Primary Care: Core values

Primary Care: Core values

Edited by

MIKE PRINGLE
Professor, Division of General Practice,
Queens Medical Centre,
Nottingham, UK

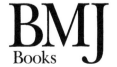

First published in 1998
by BMJ Books, BMA House, Tavistock Square,
London WC1H 9JR

British Library Cataloguing in Publication Data

A catalogue record for this book is available from the British Library

ISBN 0-7279-1268-2

Typeset by Apek Typesetters, Nailsea, Bristol
Printed and bound by Latimer Trend, Plymouth.

Contents

Contributors

Jennifer Dixon
Fellow in Health Policy Analysis
Kings Fund
11-13 Cavendish Square, London, UK

Brian M Goss
General Practitioner
Beeches, Bungay, Suffolk, UK

Jacky Hayden
Dean of Postgraduate Medicine
The University of Manchester, Department of Postgraduate
Medicine and Dentistry, Gateway House, Piccadilly South,
Manchester, UK

Iona Heath
General Practitioner,
Caversham Group Practice, Kentish Town Health Centre,
2 Batholomew Road, London, UK

Peter Holland
Associate Director,
Lambeth Southwark and Lewisham Health Authority,
1 Lower Marsh, London, UK

Nicholas Mays
Director of Health Services Research,
King's Fund, 11-13 Cavendish Square, London, UK

Ian R McWhinney
Professor Emeritus
Centre for Studies in Family Medicine, Department of Family
Medicine, The University of Western Ontario, London, Canada

Rabbi Julia Neuberger
Chief Executive
King's Fund, 11-13 Cavendish Square, London, UK

John Roberts
Staff Physician, Madrona Medical Group, 4465 Cordata Parkway,
Bellingham, Washington 98226, USA

Les Toop
Pegasus Professor of General Practice,
Department of General Practice, Christchurch School of Medi-
cine, Otago University Medical School, Christchurch, New
Zealand

Chris Van Weel
Professor of General Practice,
Department of General Practice and Social Medicine,
University of Nijmegen, PO Box 9101, 6500 HB Nijmegen,
The Netherlands

Preface

Depending on your perspective, these are times of excitement or trauma in primary care. For all of us they cannot fail to be interesting. Fundamental changes in health service planning, organisation and delivery are occurring worldwide and, fascinatingly and significantly, are pointing in the same direction of travel.

Medicine in the last century can be characterised as pastoral. Therapeutic interventions, except for those which had persisted through from the hebalism of previous centuries, were often ill-informed, brutal and risky. With the advent of scientific medicine hospital based care developed throughout the first half of this century in industrialised countries, and has been transferred to the less developed world through the empires.

There has been, however, a clear shift in the second half of the twentieth century. The effectiveness of secondary care interventions has increased, but their costs have escalated to beyond the means of most societies. Concentrating massive health resources on increasingly fewer individuals has raised a political and ethical debate.

Beside this debate lies one of far greater significance for primary care, for it is a debate about values. We can all imagine the care we might wish for if we were, for example, diagnosed as having a cancer. We would, of course, wish for high quality technical care in treating the tumour and giving us the greatest chance of survival.

However we would also wish for prevention and screening services, giving us the best chance of avoiding the cancer and of picking it up at an early, treatable stage. We would want to be told of the diagnosis in an humane manner and to have a knowledgeable and caring health professional travelling through the illness beside us. We would wish to be able to share our hopes and fears, to have an understanding of the process of the disease and its care, and to be an equal partner in decisions that intimately involve our health.

And when death comes near, we would want to be in familiar surroundings free, as far as possible, from fear and pain, supported by our family and friends - the latter including our health professionals.

These are not the aspirations only of doctors. These are the aspirations of all our patients. For many reasons - the suddenness of the death, the specific dimensions of the illness - these aspirations cannot be met; yet we should strive to achieve them whenever possible.

These characteristics are, quintessentially, those of primary care. We rely heavily on colleagues in other sectors of the health service to provide technical care, and many doctors and nurses in hospital settings offer long term personal commitment to patients. Yet, wherever they are exercised, these features represent the value system of primary care and, in Britain, have been encapsulated into the concept of a "Primary Care Led NHS".

Worldwide, societies are trying to create health services that offer them the care that they really want at a price that they can afford. These economic and value-driven agendas make for some difficult, uncomfortable choices. Increasingly, however, governments are confronting those choices and moving towards services based on a primary care foundation.

In the dark days it has been all too easy to lose faith in the core values of primary care. But they survived because they are robust and are right. In this book a range of eminent authors reflect on those core values and their relevance to the development of health services today. As we refashion our health services we must emphasise the strengths of primary care and ensure that the delivery of health meets the aspirations of patients, societies and those of us who work in health care.

Mike Pringle

1 Core values in a changing world

Ian R McWhinney

In 1920, the Dawson report advocated a population based approach to the organisation of health services, the allocation of resources, and the training of health care staff.[1] It also introduced the concepts of primary and secondary levels of care and of primary care health centres. For several decades these ideas lay dormant, until medical specialisation, fragmentation of health services, and the introduction of publicly funded health care made their logic inescapable. The term "primary care" became common coinage, and in 1978 its fundamental importance was recognised by the World Health Organisation.[2] In the same year, the US Institute of Medicine identified the four essentials of good primary care as accessibility, comprehensiveness, coordination, and continuity.[3]

For most of this century, the typical primary care professional has been a generalist practitioner,[4] usually practising close to the population served by the practice, alone or in a small group, and supported by a small staff. (Generalist practitioners include practitioners from nursing and from general paediatrics or internal medicine.) The key relationship for most of these practitioners is with individual patients who consult about problems they have identified themselves. Until recently, screening for risk factors and early disease in asymptomatic patients has been unusual. But practitioners have often forged strong community links, especially in small towns and rural areas. For all its limitations, generalist practice has represented a strong tradition of personal care, comprehensive in its response to the needs of the people and reasonably accessible in their neighbourhoods and homes. It is on this living tradition that primary care should build as it evolves into new forms.

Traditions are the bearers of values. In a living tradition, there is a perennial debate about how the inherent goods of the tradition are to be realised. The debate takes on a special poignancy when there is a conflict between one good and another. Alastair

1

Macintyre distinguishes between the internal and external goods of traditional practices and institutions.[5] The external goods are those for which the insitituion competes, such as prestige, money, market share, power. The internal goods are those that enable members of the institution to practise in accordance with their ideals and to attain fulfillment in their work. Conflicts between these two goods are a perennial issue for all traditions. The relentless pursuit of one good can destroy the other and ultimately bring down the whole institution. The continuing strength of a tradition is the best assurance that these conflicting goods will be reconciled.

The practitioner and the patient

Traditionally, the commitment of the generalist practitioner is to the person, not to "the person with a certain disease." General practice defines itself in terms of relationships, not in terms of diseases or technologies. The commitment is open ended. The relationship is ended only by retirement, removal, death, or a decision by either party to end it.

The key role of the generalist practitioner is responding to the initial presentation of illness, through responding to suffering and making a clinical assessment. How events unfold is profoundly influened by this initial response. Responding to suffering is a moral obligation. Compassion is not, as some have suggested, conditional on evidence of its effectiveness.[6] Although a practitioner or a practice may enter into a contract with a paying agency, the relationship with a patient is better described as a covenant.[7] A contract sets out the limits of what can be expected of the parties. It says: "I am committed to doing so much, but not more." A covenant is an undertaking to do whatever is needed, even if it goes beyond the terms of the contract. Sticking with a person through thick and thin is hard work: an act of love, not in the affective sense, but in Dostoevsky's sense of active love: "hard work and tenacity and for some people perhaps . . . a whole science".[8]

The healing relationship between practitioner and patient can take its place beside others in which there are strong moral obligations and mutual commitments, such as those between parent and child and teacher and student. Although continuity is important in all of them, it is not simply a matter of chronological time. There are inevitable breaks of continuity in any relationship. No practitioner can be available to patients at all times. A good relationship, however, requires continuity of responsibility. Responsible practitioners will want to provide a deputy who can give care as close as possible to the care they can provide, and they will want to be present at times of great need. We seem almost to have forgotten the importance in medicine of presence. Of course, this faces us with many conflicting moral choices between obligations to different patients, to our families, and to ourselves.

Continuity in relationships builds trust, creates a context for healing, and increases the practitioner's knowledge of the patient, much of it at the tacit level.[9] Since it concerns responsibility and commitment, it is a moral issue for practitioners of all professions in primary care, and for their patients. A relationship with one doctor is strongly preferred by most patients and doctors, but some patients view it as continuity with a practice, and others give a higher value to accessibility.[10] Patients can have strong feelings of continuing care from a familiar doctor, practice nurse, and receptionist working together.[11] The preconditions of continuity are ready access, competence of the doctor, good communication, and a mechanism for bridging from one consultation to the next.[10] Continuity is a mutual commitment by patient and practitioner.[9,10] A practitioner's sense of responsibility increases with the duration of the relationship and with the number of contacts.[9]

Obstacles to continuity

Some obstacles to continuity, such as long distance commuting and population mobility, are features of modern industrial societies. Others lie in the management of the health care system, in communication between primary and secondary sectors, in management of the practice, and in the operations of the primary care team.

Management's drive for efficiency can threaten relationships by rigidly defining professional roles and by penalising practitioners who step outside their role. No doubt it is inefficient for a doctor to attend to an old person's callosities and toenails, but it is through such little services that relationships are built. Some doctors and nurses may have special expertise in managing asthma, diabetes, or advanced cancer, but this does not mean that every one of these patients has to be transferred to their care. A patient's relationship with the primary care practitioner may be broken if there is poor coordination between primary, secondary, and tertiary care sectors. The organisation of a practice may itself be an impediment to continuity.

Relationships with colleagues

Teamwork enhances primary care, but it requires wise leadership, attention to team relationships, and a change in traditional professional values. The growth of teams has been rapid in the past two decades as doctors and nurses have often been joined by social workers, psychologists, counsellors, physiotherapists, and pharmacists. Breaks in continuity, poor coordination, and blurring of responsibility are among the faults attributed to the primary care team.

The evolving nurse-doctor relationship is the key to the future of primary care. Each profession has its central role, but there is much overlap, and the roles should be allowed to evolve over time with minimal direction. The value of teamwork is in the diverse perspectives of the professions. From their integration emerges a new level of care, different from each of the individual perspectives. We have so much to learn from each other, but we can only learn if we approach teamwork with what Wilber calls an aperspectival frame of mind.[12] This means valuing all perspectives, but regarding none as final – not even our own. It requires in us a capacity to step out of our own perspective and to view it from outside, as we view those of others. In the same way, the patient-centred clinical method aims to integrate the perspectives of doctor and patient.[13] "No perspective is final," however, is not the same as the moral relativism of "all perspectives are equal".

In a well functioning team the members meet together regularly, learn from each other, and care for each other as well as for their patients. When discussions about patients result in decisions, the responsibility for implementation is clearly defined. Whether it is alongstanding team or one assembled for a particular patient, a team needs a leader. Leadership should be open to any of the practitioners in the team. This is difficult if some team members are in an employer-employee relationship.

Clinical freedom and managed care

The freedom to practice in accordance with the highest standards is highly valued by all professions. Constraints are always present, but clinical freedom allows practitioners the flexibility to

4

make difficult choices between competing priorities. The choices may range from decisions about how much time to spend with a particular patient to the allocation of the practice's resources among preventive, clinical, and managerial functions. With this freedom goes the moral obligation to do everything needed for the individual patient and to use the least resources necessary to attain this end. Family physicians are notable for their restraint in using resources without impairing the quality of care.[14] At the same time they strongly resist measures designed to limit services at the point of care in the name of efficiency. To clinicians, efficacy – and not efficiency – has the higher value.

Under managed care in its various forms, restrictions on clinicians have now become commonplace. Modern information systems make it possible for managers to monitor and control practitioners' behaviour by such measures as utilisation review, incentives and disincentives, and preauthorisation for procedures and referrals. This is so destructive of professional morale that it may become self defeating. If limits to resources are established by society they can be subject to public scrutiny. The transfer of financial risk to practitioners gives practices the freedom to make their own decisions about the distribution of resources. Self-imposed limits are more tolerable than those imposed from above, but if we stand to gain from the decisions ourselves, our interests are potentially in conflict with those of our patients.[15]

The practice and the community

The population perspective, ensuring that the services of the practice are made available to the whole practice population, has a long tradition in general practice.[16] Information technology has made it easier to maintain the necessary records. But if a practice is going to offer preventive services for asymptomatic patients it must ensure that such services are strongly supported by evidence.[17] The population perspective is also an attitude of mind, a looking beyond the individual patient with head injury, lead poisoning, or salmonella infection to other people at risk from the same health hazards.

Community oriented primary care takes this perspective a step further through systematically identifying health problems in the community, modifying practice procedures, and monitoring the impact of changes.[18,19,20] Such care is said to require a new kind of hybrid practitioner with competencies in primary care, prevention, epidemiology, ethics, and behavioural science. These roles may be conflicting, competing for time and resources and causing tension in individual practitioners and practices. For the practitioner, community oriented primary care could usurp essential clinical skills. However, the principles of such care can be applied in other ways, such as by collaboration between all practices in a community or geographical locality for purposes such as deputising arrangements, hospital discharge planning, or shared care schemes. A group of community practices could also collaborate with a health unit or social agency to address problems such as homelessness, child poverty, and malnutrition. The Divisions of General Practice in Australia are moving in this direction.[21] In Britain, general practitioners are, increasingly, working together in locality groups, rather than as individual fundholders. They commission (and sometimes purchase) the secondary care that their communities, based on local epidemiology and needs assessment. New legislation will oblige all general practitioners, from 1999, to work together in large primary care groups. These will work with health authorities and local authorities to commission all health care.

The human scale

General practice has traditionally been carried on in small units located close to the homes of patients. Primary care should continue this tradition, continuing to be accessible to patients and avoiding the anonymity and intimidating atmosphere that tends to go with larger institutions. Embedding the practice in the community that it serves helps the staff to form links with the community and to learn about its resources.

I thank Thomas Freeman, Joseph Morrissy, and Wayne Weston for their helpful suggestions, and Bette Cunningham for preparing the manuscript.

1 White KL. Historical preface. In: Lamberts H, Wood M, eds. *International Classification of Primary Care*. Oxford: Oxford University Press, 1987.
2 World Health Organisation. *Alma-Ata 1978: primary health care*. Geneva: World Health Organisation, 1978.
3 Institute of Medicine, Division of Health Manpower and Resources Development. *Report of a study: a manpower policy for primary health care*. Washington, DC: National Academy of Sciences; 1978. (IOM publication 73-02.)
4 Carmichael LP. The GP is back. Am Family Physician 1997;56:713–4.
5 Macintyre A. *After virtue: a study in moral theory*. London: Duckworth, 1981.
6 Evidence-based Medicine Working Group. Evidence-based medicine: a new approach to the teaching the practice of medicine. *JAMA* 1992;268:2420–5.

7 May WF. *The physician's covenant — images of the healer in medical ethics*. Philadelphia: Westminster Press, 1983.

8 Dostoevsky F. *The brothers Karamazov*. Harmondsworth: Penguin, 1958. (Translated by D Magarshack.)

9 Hjortdahl R. Continuity of care: general practitioners' knowledge about, and sense of responsibility towards their patients. *Fam Pract* 1992;**9**:3–8.

10 Veale BM. Continuity of care and general practice utilisation in Australia [dissertation]. Canberra: Australian National University, 1996.

11 Brown JB, Dickie I, Brown L, Biehn J. Factors contributing to the longterm attendance of patients at a family practice teaching unit. *Can Fam Physician* 1997;**43**:901–6.

12 McWhinney IR. Caring for patients with cancer: family physicians' role. *Can Fam Physician* 1994;**40**:16–7.

13 Wilber K. *Sex, ecology and spirituality*. Boston: Shambhala, 1995.

14 Stewart M, Brown JB, Weston WW, McWhinney IR, Freeman TR, et al. *Patient-centred medicine*. Newbury Park, CA: Sage, 1995.

15 Franks P, Clancy CM, Nutting PA. Gatekeeping revisited — protecting patients from overtreatment. *N Engl J Med* 1992;**327**:424–9.

16 Smith LFP, Morrissy JR. Ethical dilemmas for general practitioners under the new UK contract. *J Med Ethics* 1994;**20**:175–80.

17 Hart JT. Semicontinuous screening of a whole community for hypertension. *Lancet* 1970;**2**:223.

18 McCormick J. Health promotion: the ethical dimension. *Lancet* 1994;**344**:390–1.

19 Nutting PA. Community-oriented primary care: an integrated model for practice, research, and education. *Am J Prev Med* 1986;**2**:140–7.

20 Nutting PA, Connor EM. Community-oriented primary care: an examination of the US experience. *Am J Public Health* 1986;**76**:279–81.

21 Wright RA. Community-oriented primary care. *JAMA* 1993;**269**:2544–7.

22 Saltman DC. Divisions of general practice: too much too quickly. *Med J Aust* 1995;**162**:3–4.

2 Patient-centred primary care

Les Toop

In this chapter, Les Toop, recently appointed to the Chair of General Practice in Christchurch, New Zealand, reflects on the evolving nature of the relationships between patients and clinicians – doctors, nurses and others – working in primary care. After considering internal pressure on the consultation, largely derived from changing expectations, and external pressures from changes in society, he espouses the *sustained partnership* model of interaction and a viable paradigm for the clinician-patient relationship of the future.

Introduction

The importance and primacy of the clinician-patient relationship cannot be overstated. This relationship's perceived intrinsic quality initially allows two individuals, previously unknown to each other, to feel comfortable with an often high level of intimacy. With time the relationship may develop to allow safe and constructive discussion of intensely personal and private matters. The bond that forms may be healing in and of itself.[1] However, the changing expectations of both clinicians and patients, together with changes to the context in which the interactions take place, challenge the future of this relationship.

In this chapter, the generic term *clinician* has been chosen deliberately to reflect the increasing variety of health professionals – not just doctors – now involved in providing primary health care to individuals in the community.[2] The term *patient* has been retained for want of a better one.[3]

Pressures from within the consultation

The way the clinician and the patient relate to each other is a major determinant of the outcomes of a consultation. Satisfaction for both[4] and degree of patients' compliance with management

8

plans[5] are directly related to the quality of various elements of the clinician-patient relationship. We know much less about the effects of the relationship on measurable health outcomes.

What are the desirable elements of this relationship between clinician and patient and how might these change in the future? Ian McWhinney describes the relationship between clinician and patient as one of open ended commitment on the part of the clinician, a covenant going well beyond the boundaries of any contract with a purchaser of health services.[2] He emphasises the importance of both the human and the healing relationships which develop between practitioners and patients, along with the need to provide continuity of responsibility, even if practitioners cannot always be there for patients.[2]

We do not know how many patients want such a covenant. Many clinicians strive to deliver it with various levels of success and at varying costs to themselves and those around them. Expectations are changing and the differences between the two ends of the spectrum, from the traditional practice to the one-stop McHealthcare, are widening. Caring for a diverse population is becoming increasingly complex. The generalist has to cater for an ever widening range of patient expectations and develop the skills needed to switch between styles of interaction.

Alongside the changing expectations of patients are those of the clinicians. Is vocation strong and enduring enough to survive the demands of increased expectations of patients, of the system and the competing claims and obligations to self and to family? Judging by the recent difficulties of recruitment and retention to general practice in Britain it would seem that the scales are tipping, and for many the answer is "no".

Organisational changes

Increased teamwork in primary care should help, in theory, by sharing the burden of responsibility and, in some contexts, on call commitments. However, teamwork may also blur responsibility and reduce personal care. For many, development and extension of the core primary care team of nurses and doctors working collaboratively offers the way for the future.[2] Such development might necessitate more shared multidisciplinary education and training.

In some places this teamwork approach already exists, seems to work well and is very acceptable to the users. The potential number of disciplines who might claim to be part of the extended (as opposed to the core) primary care team seems to have no boundaries. Clearly, above a certain size the transaction time and costs of trying to work as a cohesive team are prohibitive.[3] There is a danger that managing team function and structure becomes an end in itself and, as a result, the needs of patients become secondary to the process.

Lack of time has become one of the catchphrases of healthcare in the 80s and 90s. How can constructive, efficient, caring and healing relationships be built up with more than a thousand individuals in a series of short and intermittent general practice consultations punctuated by constant interruption and coloured by anticipatory stress of further work commitments? John Howie's work has shown the effects of consultation time on doctors' levels of stress and on patient empowerment.[6] There will always be tension between the unpredictable quantum of time needed by individual patients and the competing need to run a system efficient enough to allow patients and clinicians to at least start their interaction in a positive and relaxed frame of mind.

Societal pressures on the consultation

There are of course many other external influences which may cause problems with the clinician-patient relationship. In many countries legislation on privacy and confidentiality can cause problems with access to health information and to effective teamwork. In a recent survey in New Zealand the public were completely divided about who should have access to general practitioners' records: at one extreme respondents expected access to be restricted to one person only (i.e. not even a locum), whereas at the liberal end people thought anyone involved, however peripherally, with their care could see the records.[7]

Many countries have also enacted legislation on consumer information and protection. Is it always possible for consumers of health care to be fully informed? Concepts such as relative and absolute risk, number needed to treat, cost effectiveness and resource allocation might not always be explainable to patients, yet these concepts are clearly important in making informed choices. Trying to juggle advocacy for individual patients with decisions on resource allocation for wide society leaves clinicians with conflicting moral obligations.

10

The sustained partnership

The positive value of a strong, trusting and lasting relationship between clinician and patient is as important as ever. Numerous models have been proposed to describe the types of clinician-patient relationship. Twenty years ago Szasz and Hollender described three basic models[8]: the *activity-passivity* approach based on the parent-infant model; the *guidance cooperation* approach based on the parent-child; and the *mutual participation* based on the adult-adult interaction. In the latter the doctor helps the patient to help themselves and the patient is a participant in the "partnership".

None of these three is claimed to be better than the others; each have their place and each may be inappropriate at times. Too many doctors may be stuck in the guidance-cooperation model and feel that their authority is threatened if patients are allowed too much autonomy and too great a share of the executive role.[9]

The patient-centred approach (based on mutual participation) has gained increasing support in recent years.[10] This approach reaches a shared acceptance of the agreed roles of the clinician and patient, of the nature and extent of the patient's problem, and of the goals each has for the interaction. Equally important is shared responsibility for achieving the agreed goals. There is not yet, however, any solid evidence that patient centred care improves health outcomes.

In 1994 the US Institute of Medicine included in its definition of primary care the concept of a *sustained partnership* between patient and clinician.[4]. While denoting participation from both parties, this concept does not necessarily imply equal roles. This concept has been picked up by Nancy Leopold and colleagues who have developed an attractive model for this sustained partnership (see Box 2.1).[11] The defining features of this model are: whole person focus; doctor's knowledge of patient; caring and empathy; trust; choice of appropriately adapted care; and finally, patient participation and shared decision-making. It is a moot point whether one clinician ever could or would provide all of this. In primary care teams embodying true collaboration and shared ownership such a model of sustained partnership should be developed through a successful triad of relationships, founded between the doctor, the nurse and the patient.

Box 2.1 Sustained Partnership. Defining Features (Leopold et al[11])

1 *Whole person focus.* The physician attends "to all health-related problems, either directly or through collaboration, regardless of the nature, origin, or organ system affected" (Safran DG. Unpublished background paper written for the Institution of Medicine's interim report of 1994[1]).

2 *Physician's knowledge of the patient.* The physician knows not just the patient's medical history, but his or her personal history, family, work, and community and cultural context, as well as his or her preferences, values, beliefs, and ideals about health care, including preferences for information and participation in clinical decision-making.

3 *Caring and empathy.* The physician expresses humaneness toward the patient through such qualities as interest, concern, compassion, sympathy, empathy, attentiveness, sensitivity, and consideration.

4 *Patient trust of physician.* The patient believes that the physician's words and actions are credible and reliable, that the physician will act in the patient's best interest based on the physician's clinical knowledge and knowledge of the patient, and that the physician will provide support and assistance concerning treatment and medical care.

5 *Appropriately adapted care.* The physician tailors treatment recommendations to reflect the patient's goals and expectations regarding health and health care as well as the patient's beliefs, values, and life circumstances.

6 *Patient participation and shared decision-making.* The physician encourages the patient to participate in all aspects of care, and treatment and referrals are agreed to by both physician and patient. To the extent that the patient wishes, the physician informs the patient about diagnosis, prognosis, and treatment options and includes the patient in treatment decisions.

Conclusions

Despite being so central to the discipline of medicine, the clinician-patient relationship is under attack from within through evolving expectations of both parties - and from outside, through changing norms in society. Models of the consultation in which the doctor maintains a more mature, and controlling, role than the patient have persisted through to the present day. The doctor of the future, however, will find that such models are increasingly unacceptable, particulary in primary care. The sustained partnership model ensures a patient-centred relationship that does not devalue special skills of the clinician.

Acknowledgements

My thanks to Jean Ross for helpful comments on the manuscript.

1. Donaldson M. Yordy K, Vanselow N eds.Institute of Medicine. *Defining primary care:an interim report.* Washington DC: National Academy Press, 1994: pp.20-1.
2. Royal College of General Practitioners *The nature of general medical practice. RCGP* 1996.
3. Probert CSJ, Battock T, Mayberry JF. Consumer, customer, client or patient. *Lancet* 1990; **335**: 1446-7.
4. Hjortdahl P, Laerum E. Continuity of care in general practice: effect on patient satisfaction. *Br Med J* 1992;**304**:1287-90.
5. Frank K, Kupfer DJ, Siegel LR. Alliance not compliance: a philosophy of outpatient care. *J Clin Psychiatry* 1995; **56** (suppl):11-17.
6. Howie J, Porter M, Heaney D. General practitioners, work and stress. In: Royal College of General Practitioners *Stress management in general practice* London: RCGP, 1993 (occasional paper 61.)
7. Toop LJ, Hodges I. *What level of primary care teamwork does the New Zealand population want? (in press)*
8. Szasz TS, Hollender MH. The Basic Models of the Doctor-Patient Relationship. *Arch Intern Med* 1976;**97**:585-9.
9. Lawrence SL. The physician's perception of health care. *J R Soc Med* 1994; **22**:11-14.
10. Stewart M, Brown JB, Weston WW, McWhinney IR, Freeman TR, McWilliam CL. *Patient-Centred Medicine.* Newbury Park, CA Sage Publications: 1995.
11. Leopold N, Cooper J, Clancy C. Sustained Partnership in Primary Care. *J am Pract* 1996; **42**:129-137.

3 Contracting for general practice: another turn of the wheel of history

Brian M Goss

The current British debate concerning funding for the health service and, thus, the nature of the general practitioner contract, is the subject of this chapter by Brian Goss, a GMSC negotiator from 1992–1997. In recognising the fact that the general practitioner has always earned income from multiple sources and has adapted to historical circumstances, he signposts new developments in the general practice contract. While an essentially parochial review, the underlying messages in this chapter are relevant to general practitioners and policy-makers internationally.

Déjà vu

British general practitioners often assert their pride at being "independent contractors", without remembering the origin of the term. Dr Ransome, pictured on his rounds as visiting physician to the local cottage hospital (Figure 3.1), was one of my predecessors in practice, and his extract from Kelly"s 1908 directory of trade and professional people reminds us how most of our medical forbears earned their living (Box 3.1). Others of my nineteenth

---

Box 3.1 (*Kelly"s Directory of Suffolk, 1908.*)

RANSOME, Gilbert Holland. LRCP Lond, MRCS Eng. Physician & Surgeon. Medical officer and public vaccinator to Bungay District Council. Medical officer to Wangford Union and 4th District. Medical officer to Loddon and Clavering Union and 2nd District. Medical officer to Depwade Union.

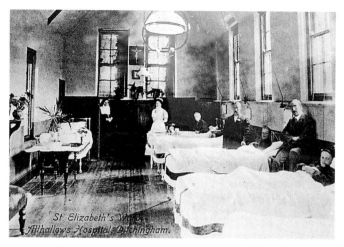

Figure 3.1 Dr Ransome at All Hallows Hospital, Ditchingham, Nr Bungay, Suffolk

century medical ancestors are entered as Surgeon to Waveney Valley Branch of Great Eastern Railway (Dr Adams, 1875[1]), Surgeon to the Dispensary for the Poor (Dr Garneys, 1828[2]), and Surgeon to the Rational Sick and Burial Association (Dr Johnstone, 1890[3]).

This collection of contracts included occupational and public health services, treatment and certification of subscribers to friendly societies, care of inpatients at cottage hospitals and a very basic service to the indigent poor, whether inside workhouses (Figure 3.2) or on "outdoor relief", as the forerunner of social security payment was called.

Although these arrangements initially seem to be relics of a bygone age, the modern general practitioner who immunises children and adults, sees patients at the surgery or in the home, visits residential homes, and has hospital practitioner contracts at a community hospital or in a district hospital specialist department, has a spectrum of work that bears a remarkable resemblance to that of Dr Ransome and his Victorian colleagues.

As well as these contracts these doctors would, of course, have undertaken private consulting practice. John Scott, a well-to-do local diarist, records that he consulted Dr Garneys about his feeble sister Charlotte[2], and, on behalf of concerned local worthies, about the 1849 outbreak of cholera in the town[4]. On New Year"s Eve

15

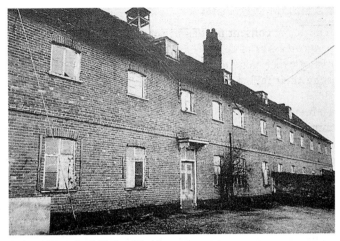

Figure 3.2   Wangford Union Workhouse

1828 Dr Garneys was even called upon to "dissect" Scott's gardener, James Baker, who died of "Billious (sic) Fever and Metastasis .... leading to congestion of the brain"[2].

General practice in the NHS

The NHS arose from the atmosphere of social cohesion and unity of national purpose which developed during the Second World War. It is neatly expressed by the famous "Assumption B" of the Beveridge report[8], which gave rise to the NHS:

> That a comprehensive national health service will ensure that for every citizen there is available whatever medical treatment he requires, in whatever form he requires it, domiciliary or institutional, general, specialist, or consultant, and will ensure also the provision of dental, ophthalmic, and surgical appliances, nursing and midwifery, and rehabilitation after accidents.[6]

After the foundation of the NHS in 1948 general practitioners became used to receiving ever higher proportions of their gross income from NHS sources. As Julian Tudor Hart recalled:

> I qualified [in 1952] and will retire from full-time clinical practice in 1988; the NHS allowed me to do my own work and refer my patients to the whole range of specialist services during an entire working lifetime, without ever having to collect a fee. Several generations of British doctors have followed, with essentially the same historically novel experience.[5]

16

End of the NHS era

The social consent needed to fully fund a comprehensive NHS, free at the point of delivery can, I fear, no longer be relied upon - a reality which general practitioners may be the last to recognise, despite their falling income against comparator professions since 1980.

Neither of the two major political parties in Britain has committed itself to raising taxation in order to increase spending on the NHS and other public services. The public has shown increasing tolerance of erosions at important margins of the NHS over the past three decades (under both right and left wing governments) including the progressive partial privatisation of care of the elderly, optical services and dental services, the private finance initiative, and enormous leaps in prescription charges, all tolerated without political damage. Public consent for privatisation is not expressed through lack of commitment to the NHS, which is highly valued, but through a reluctance to accept the increased taxation which is necessary to deliver Beveridge"s "Assumption B".

The public is also willing to pay for supplementary health services and products including burgeoning publications and telephone advice lines on health, private general practice on demand in railway stations and other locations, a steadily increasing market in over-the-counter medicines, and private elective surgery. On the other hand, compared to other developed countries, the UK still has a strikingly low proportion of private health spending.

A mixed economy between NHS and private work is accepted by many dentists and consultants as part of their traditional pattern of work. This does not sit so easily with general practitioners, however, who are inhibited from mixing NHS and private work for the same patient not only by philosophical inclination, but by their terms of service.

Despite this, general practitioners in the closing years of the century may have to bring a higher and more flexible proportion of private funding into general practice, given that the opportunities and political will to invest in the NHS from public sources seems increasingly limited.

Recognising general practitioners' limits

General practitioners, on the whole, remain fiercely committed to a comprehensive NHS. Yet recent developments in general practice signify their willingness to recognise the personal and professional limits of doctors" ability to meet the quantity and nature of demand, in a way that would have been unthinkable a decade ago.

Following a crisis in out of hours primary care in 1995[7], doctors, patients and government alike recognised that a service based entirely on home visits could not satisfy rising demand within existing financial constraints. Consequently, and with modest additional funding from the government, general practitioners began to offer out of hours care at primary care premises, and to work together in cooperatives covering larger areas and larger populations[8].

At around the same time general practitioners demanded set limits on the scope of their practice[9]. This arose mainly from the considerable shift of work from the secondary to primary care sector, without shifted funding, following the internal market reforms of 1990.

The publication of a clear definition of core general practice in 1996[9] allowed family doctors to draw a line in the sand, demarcating the myriad small tasks farmed out from hospitals, and the care of patients sent to nursing homes who would, formerly, have occupied places in long stay hospitals.

General practitioners have responded to the definition of core services in a variety of ways. Some have been keen to take additional training to contract for new non-core tasks or care for more complex groups of patients under supplementary contracts. Others have insisted that they do not wish to undertake the work even under contract. The 1997 Primary Care Act[10] opened up further contractual possibilities for general practitioners. General practice can now be provided under a contract made by health authorities with a trust or group of practitioners, instead of having to be provided under the traditional and highly regulated environment of part 2 of the 1977 NHS Act. In the new style of practice, patients will register with the Trust rather than with an individual doctor, and responsibility will be held by the organisation. The employed doctors will have contractual responsibilities to their employers. This model has been further encouraged by the Labour government's White Paper, *The New NHS – modern, dependable*, which encourages doctors to move towards primary care trusts status.

The future of contracts

The future general practitioner will probably have a wide network of contracts. As resources fail to expand to meet demand the NHS contract for general practice may be increasingly focused on the poorest and most deprived patients, leaving the better off to make private provision from the proceeds of a low tax economy.

General practitioners with wide ranging skills and interests may, however, contract to care for specialised groups in nursing and residential homes, to provide surgical services and procedures within their practices, to perform occupational health examinations and advice, to provide services to a corporate provider in the primary health care business, and, eventually, to contract individually with private patients.

Whatever general practitioners do, they always need to remember the nature of their core business. The following words from an early draft of the BMA"s statement on core services encapsulate what GPs are best at, and what they see as their central expertise, regardless of whether the funding comes from public, private or mixed sources:

> The irreducible essence of general practice is the care of people who are or believe themselves to be ill. Sensing unease within themselves which is not resolved using their own perceptions or the resources of those around them, people seek a consultation to secure an understanding of what is happening to them, what it means and what might be done with what effect. This aspect of human behaviour transcends history, geography and culture and will survive the ephemeral health policies of transient governments. Providing a response to these concerns is what most general practitioners feel they are best at and are happiest doing. By identifying the heart of our craft as the response to this timeless human need, we at a stroke restate our *raison d"être* and define our sovereign professional territory at a time of doubt and demoralisation.[11]

Adapt or perish

Sadly, the public's aversion to taxation means that general practitioners are still prone to the sort of pressure and exploitation in the public service that Punch magazine satirised a century and a half ago (Figure 3.3), and which survives today in the form of the Doctors and Dentists Review Body. The survival of personal medicine requires, as it always has done, imaginative adaptation by doctors to the economic and social realities that surround the timeless human need for access to healers.

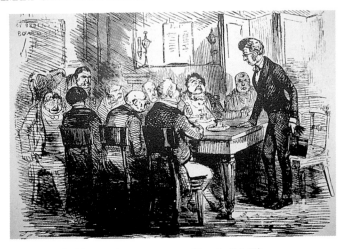

Figure 3.3   Workhouse doctor cartoon, Punch (1848)

Chairman : "Well, young man. So you wish to be engaged as parish doctor?"

Doctor : "Yes, gentlemen, I am desirous -"

Chairman : "Ah! Exactly. Well, it's understood that your wages - salary I should say - is to be twenty pounds per annum; and you find your own tea and sugar - medicines I mean - and, in fact, make yourself generally useful. If you do your duty, and conduct yourself properly, why - ah - you - ah -"

(*Punch* : "Will probably be bowled out of your situation by some humbug who will fill it for less money.")

Splendid opening for a young medical man. Punch (1848).

1. Kelly"s Directory of Suffolk, 1875.
2. Scott, J B, In Ethel Mann, Ed. *"An Englishman at Home and Abroad 1792-1828"*, Bungay Morrow & Co: 1988, page 217.
3. Rayner"s Bungay Almanac 1890.
4. Scott, J B, In Ethel Mann and Hugh Cane, Eds. Bungay, Morrow & Co: 1996 p 160.
5. Hart, J T, *"A New Kind of Doctor"*, Merlin, 1988.
6. Report on Social Insurance and Allied Services. Sir William Beveridge. HMSO, 1942, Cmd 6404.
7. Heath, I. General Practice at Night. *Br Med J* 1995;**311**:466.
8. Jessopp, L, Beck, I, Hollins, L, Shipman, C, Reynolds, M, Dale, J. Changing the pattern of out of hours care: a survey of general practice cooperatives. *Br Med J* 1997;**314**:199–200.
9. Core Services: Taking the initiative, GMSC, 1996.
10. National Health Service (Primary Care) Act, HMSO, 1997.
11. *"Core General Medical Services and the classification of General Practitioner Activity"*, Appendix II, GMSC Annual Report, 1995, GMSC 1995.

4 Developing primary care: gatekeeping, commissioning, and managed care

Jennifer Dixon, Peter Holland, Nicholas Mays

The people and structures who make up the NHS in the UK have shown remarkable flexibility over the past 50 years. In the past decade, particularly, primary care has taken on a whole new set of responsibilities: commissioning and purchasing care for local populations.

In this chapter Dixon, Holland and Mays explain the latest changes for general practitioners and others in primary care and suggest the future challenges for this key part of the NHS

If Nye Bevan were around today, he might be surprised to find that the basic features of British general practice, not least its administrative separation from hospital care, are still in place half a century after the genesis of the NHS. But, of course, primary care has not stood still over that period - both its structure and role have developed continuously.

This development has not been part of an orchestrated grand plan. Rather, it has been characterised by incremental change in response to wider pressures. For example, new technologies have allowed more treatment at home and shorter lengths of stay in hospital. Patients' expectations have risen about being treated promptly, and at, or close to, home. Professional expectations of primary care staff, particularly general practitioners, have moved towards wanting greater flexibility and choice in their roles at work and in their longer term careers. Underlying all of these pressures has been the increasing imperative to curb health care expenditure, contain demands, and increase efficiency. This imperative has led to a new responsibility for primary care professionals in the NHS - purchasing or commissioning secondary care.

In this chapter we examine briefly how some of these pressures have recently influenced the shape and direction of primary care in the UK, and reflect upon the direction of further change in future.

Pressures influencing the shape of primary care

Of the pressures outlined above, the greatest at present is the imperative to control the rising costs of health care. Consequently, some of the prime movers shaping the development of health systems in the UK and other countries in recent years have been payers of health care, whether public or private.

Three related changes have resulted. Firstly, there has been greater investment in, and expansion of the role of, primary care and more emphasis on its gatekeeping role. Secondly, general practitioners, and to a lesser extent other primary care staff, have been given more opportunity to shape services provided in secondary care, particularly through directly managing a budget. Thirdly, incentives and rules have been applied to providers in secondary and primary care to encourage cost-conscious behaviour, reduce inappropriate or ineffective care, and promote good quality care. Each of these aims are essential elements of managed care[1,2] and are referred to in the recent white paper *The New NHS*.[3]

Greater investment in primary care and the gatekeeping role

Unlike many other countries, the UK has developed a strong system of primary care. Firm central direction has ensured universal access to a general practitioner, a healthy balance of general practitioners to hospital doctors, and greater real growth of expenditure on family health services compared to hospital and community health services - 3.7% compared to 2.9% over the past 20 years. The solo general practitioner working out of two rooms has been replaced largely by group practice, multidisciplinary teams and multipurpose health centres. The roles of primary care staff, especially nurses, have expanded and teamwork is encouraged.[4] The two recent primary care white papers stress both the development of primary care organisations to replace the independent general practitioner, and primary care as the main locus for health care activity.[5,6] In the 1990s there has been some limited attempt to influence the services provided in general practice, for example through the national general practice contract, and this is likely to continue.

Other countries are belatedly learning the value of these types of arrangements, particularly in terms of efficiency, and are rapidly reshaping their health care systems. For example, in the US there are new incentives for doctors to train as primary care physicians and for hospitals not to train more specialists.[7] Payment scales have been adjusted to favour primary care physicians over specialists,[8] [9] reimbursement for providers has shifted from fee for service to capitation, and payers are increasingly insisting that patients seeking care make first contact with a primary care gatekeeper rather than a specialist. There is thus a worldwide push to promote investment in primary care above specialist care.[10] [11]

Greater opportunity to shape the services provided in secondary care

The underlying aim of initiatives in this area is not simply to give primary care providers greater influence over secondary care. Increasingly, the government wants to encourage greater cost control and efficiency where many key decisions relating to subsequent expenditure are made - in primary care. The NHS has done this through increasing the influence of the general practitioner, rather than other members of the primary care team, or patients.

Three overlapping developments are increasingly being pursued in the UK[3]: greater contact between general practitioners, health authority purchasers, and secondary care providers; giving general practitioners and primary care organisations direct purchasing power; and, most recently, encouraging vertical and "virtual" integration of providers in primary and secondary care.

Greater contact between general practitioners, purchasers, and secondary care providers

General practitioners and other primary care staff have always had opportunities to influence care provided by other providers. They have been able to do this informally through professional networks and formally through representation on health authorities and hospital boards.

The NHS reforms of 1991 channelled general practitioner influence into the purchasing process instead.[12] General practitioners have been encouraged to influence providers indirectly through the health authority via locality commissioning and variants such as general practitioner-led commissioning, or through the new primary care groups.[3] The existing initiatives have had some impact, particularly in developing services at the interface between primary and secondary care.[13 14 15] General practitioners who purchase care (for example through fundholding or total purchasing[16]) can influence providers directly through purchasing services directly.

The reforms in 1991 offered little to encourage greater direct links between providers in primary and secondary care, other than through purchasing, possibly because efficiency was a higher concern than quality of care. Yet these links remained and have grown, despite the incentives of the internal market and other policies such as the requirement to increase hospital productivity.[17] Hospital-at-home, shared care, and outreach schemes are widespread, and some trusts are making efforts to work jointly with general practitioners on a wide range of issues.[18] The 1997 Primary Care Act and the recent white papers for England, *The New NHS*, and Scotland, *Designed to Care*,[19] mark a break with the past because they explicitly encourage links of this kind.

Giving general practitioners/primary care organisations direct purchasing power

The general practitioner fundholding scheme introduced in 1991 and its subsequent variants - community fundholding, extended fundholding, and total purchasing - gave general practitioners the opportunity to influence secondary care providers directly and provided modest incentives to shift costly hospital care to community settings. Currently around 55% of the UK population are registered with practices operating some kind of fundholding scheme.[19]

Using hard outcome measures of efficiency, equity, effectiveness, and choice for patients, the impact of fundholding has been largely equivocal.[20 21 22 23] There may be at least five reasons why the impact on curbing costs or demands, where appropriate, has been modest. Fundholding practices, at least in the early days, may have had relatively generous budgets which provided weak incentives to scrutinise expenditure.[24] Peer review of clinical behaviour is undeveloped, and adequate information to support it is often lacking. The scope for reducing hospitalisation for elective surgery may be limited, since there is little opportunity to shift it into primary care; in any case fundholding offers no significant remuneration for taking on extra work. NHS trusts may obstruct change because they see nothing positive in greater general practitioner power for general practitioners, share no mutual sense of mission, and have strong incentives to increase hospital activity while general practitioners try to reduce it. On soft outcomes such as increasing general practitioners' sense of empowerment and ability to influence other providers, fundholding has had more obvious success.[20 25] Finally, fundholding and total purchasing organisations may be too undeveloped and weak to have had much impact.[20]

This apparent lack of impact so far, plus the higher administrative costs of devolved purchasing, raise significant questions about the future impact of different forms of purchasing or commissioning. The new primary care groups covering a population of around 100 000 (set out in *The New NHS*), which will largely replace existing forms of general practitioner purchasing and commissioning, will need considerable support and help from health authorities to develop into robust and cohesive organisations. Will they be strong enough to manage demands effectively and appropriately and persuade providers to make necessary changes? Other, more fundamental, questions also need urgent answers, such as the accountability and purchasing competence of primary care groups, and the future role of health authorities[26] - only hinted at in *The New NHS*.

Regardless of the pros and cons of existing models, greater incentives to use resources for NHS care more efficiently and manage demand must be here to stay. The current proposals seek to draw all general practitioners into the mainstream task of managing NHS resources. No one model will suit all areas, however, and the umbrella term 'primary care groups' will probably cover a wide range of different organisations.

Encouraging vertical and virtual integration

Since 1991 the NHS has tried to separate purchasers and providers, and, to some degree, push purchasing into primary care. While primary and secondary care have worked together there has been no push to merge them into one "vertically integrated" organisation, until the 1997 Primary Care Act and the recent white paper *The New NHS*.

Vertically and "virtually" integrated organisations – linking primary and secondary care – are most strongly developed in the

US (particularly in California). They have developed largely in response to the pressure to control costs, and to reduce cost-shifting between different providers.[27] Vertical integration usually comprises large networks of primary care physicians and their teams working with secondary care providers in one single organisation. The organisation receives capitated payment for patient care, bears all the financial risk, and shares the benefits of any reduced resource use (such as reduced hospitalisation) amongst employees who are thus encouraged to work towards the same broad mission. "Virtual" integration is where primary care organisations (often large networks of primary care physicians) receive capitated payment for patient care, bear the financial risk of that care, and contract with preferred secondary care providers (often entering into long term relationships) without being part of the same organisation.[27]

In the UK local vertical partnerships between hospitals and community services and primary care have developed at the interface between primary and secondary care. Examples include hospital-at-home schemes, outreach, shared care, general practitioners working in A&E departments, and community staff attached to general practices as part of the primary care team. These have developed mostly to improve the quality and seamlessness of services provided, and in response to new technologies that allow more treatment at home and easier communication with hospital. But, more recently, the potential of such partnerships to contain costs by reducing unnecessary hospital use has become more apparent and important.[28]

The 1997 Primary Care Act provided the opportunity for further vertical integration. The act allowed NHS trusts (acute or community) to employ the primary team directly, including the general practitioners, and allowed the merger of budgets for General Medical Services and Hospital and Community Health Services.[29 30 31] But the underlying aim of this legislation is not clear, for example whether it is to promote more seamless care and teamwork,[32] facilitate a shift of care from hospital into the community, ease recruitment of general practitioners and practice staff, or protect the income of NHS trusts. If a main aim is to contain costs by shifting care into the community, then there may be insufficient incentives for secondary care providers to change spots and become more primary care led. But strong and stable partnerships could develop between providers in different settings under these arrangements.

The New NHS[3] and Scotland's version, *Designed to Care*,[19] both encourage primary care staff and community trusts to team up to form a single primary care trust. Furthermore, hinted at in *The New NHS*, and more explicit in *Designed to Care*, is the possibility of primary care organisations linking up more closely with hospitals through innovative local arrangements. Possible developments include vertically integrated disease management packages (for example for chronic diseases),[33] as well as schemes to pool resources and share financial incentives to keep patients out of hospital where appropriate.

In many ways virtual integration already exists in the NHS. Through fundholding and its variants, purchasers with capitated budgets, who are also primary care providers, have entered into long term contractual relationships with other providers. This has already encouraged greater efforts to provide seamless care and curb costs. For example, many of the new total purchasing pilots have made a priority of attempting to reduce both length of stay and medical admissions where appropriate[16] in order to be able to use the resources elsewhere. Some have employed "tracker" nurses to work in provider units to encourage prompter discharge for patients,[34] and others have persuaded NHS trusts to employ specialist nurses to help manage patients with chronic disease in the community. It remains to be seen whether these schemes will be effective, or whether the new primary care groups will develop them further. This partly depends on how hospitals behave – whether they will have the primary goal of increasing inpatient activity, or whether they will develop wider roles for themselves.

More incentives and rules to improve efficiency and quality

Policies to encourage efficiency have mostly been imposed by the NHS Executive; for example the discipline of living within the means of a global budget, and achieving the targets of the Purchaser Efficiency Index[35] and cost improvement programmes. The NHS reforms of 1991 aimed to increase the incentives for efficiency at a more local level through introducing the purchaser-provider split, and, in particular, by devolving budgets to primary care.

The incentives operating locally are still weak, however, which may be one reason why purchasing appears to have had a modest impact in managing demands effectively. Health authority purchasers have few direct rewards for keeping to budget; general practitioner purchasers have more but know that overspends will be met by the host health authority without real sanction; and acute trusts have incentives to increase activity, contrary to managed care goals. While there are early signs that general practitioner fundholders and total purchasers are beginning to think about peer reviewing their colleagues, health authorities have been reluctant to investigate or act upon gross variations in clinical practice. More information is becoming available on the costs of treatments, and the effectiveness of care through the research and development initiative, yet there are few direct incentives, as well as inadequate help, to use this knowledge. Proposals in *The New NHS* are designed to strengthen scrutiny of clinical performance and variations, and make much more information on the costs and effects of treatment available. The proposed Commission for Health Improvement, the nomination of a senior professional in each primary care group who will be responsible for the quality of clinical care, and the publication of a list of reference costs for hospital treatments should improve monitoring of performance. But whether the new primary care groups will act on these initiatives depends on how far they will be supported by health authorities, who are already stretched.

Even greater scrutiny of clinical behaviour is likely if resource constraints become tighter in future, if the incentives set up by different forms of purchasing through the primary care groups do not result in demands being managed more effectively, and if patients' demands for information increase. Such scrutiny may take a more aggressive form as seen in the US, such as retrospective or prospective authorisation of care before payment, utilisation review and physician profiling, more direct financial rewards for physicians to provide high quality and cost effective care, and sanctions for physicians who do not.[36] Sanctions could include exclusion from networks of providers or purchasers. These developments raise many important questions, such as who would set the criteria for, and conduct, utilisation reviews, and what will be done about poorly performing providers.

Conclusion

Primary care will develop in response to several key pressures, as it has in the past. Growth of investment in primary care relative to secondary care will continue and the role of primary care as providers will expand. Since there will be increasing pressure to control costs and demands, the role of primary care professionals as managers of resources will increase, and there will be stronger incentives to increase efficiency. These incentives may arise through devolved forms of purchasing and commissioning, or types of vertical integration, based on shared budgets. The new primary care groups will probably take many forms. *The New NHS* does not, however, clearly explain the precise objectives of the initiatives, how they will be regulated and developed, or the role of the health authority.

These developments push the NHS into the foothills of fully formed managed care. Unless the reforms result in better management of demand and increasing quality, they may curtail the freedom of primary care professionals as providers and purchasers. Direct and powerful tools to scrutinise and control clinical behaviour may become the norm, such as utilisation review with sanctions and rewards, controlled by the health authority and possibly supported by the Commission for Health Improvement. The lesson for doctors may well be "manage or be managed". In the US some of these changes have resulted in markedly diminished control over the health care delivery system by physicians, who are described as being "still in shock,"[37] something which would, perhaps, surprise Mr Bevan.

1. Fairfield G, Hunter D, Mechanic D, Flemming Rosleff. Managed care: origins, principles, and evolution. *Br Med J* 1997;**314**:1823-6.
2. MacLeod GK. An overview of managed health care. In: Kongstvedt PR (Ed). *Essentials of managed health care.* Maryland: Aspen Publications, 1995.
3. *The New NHS.* Secretary of State for England. London: The Stationery Office Limited, 1997.
4. English T. Personal paper: Medicine in the 1990s needs a team approach. *Br Med J* 1997;**314**:661-3.
5. Secretaries of State for Health in England, Wales, and Scotland. *Choice and opportunity. Primary care: The Future.* London: HMSO, October 1996.
6. *Primary care: Delivering the future.* Secretary of State for Health for England. London: HMSO, December 1996.
7. Josefson D. New York hospitals are to be paid to train fewer doctors. *Br Med J* 1997;**314**:625.
8. Hsiao WC, Braun P, Dunn D, Becker ER, DeNicola M, Ketcham TR. Results and policy implications of the resource-based relative value study. *N Engl J M* 1988;**319**:881-8.
9. Hsaio WC, Dunn DL, Verrilli DK. Assessing the implementation of physician payment reform. *N Engl J M* 1993;**328**:928-33.
10. World Bank. *World Development Report 1993.* Investing in health. Oxford: Oxford University Press, 1993.
11. The World Health Report, 1995. *Bridging the gaps.* Report of the Director General, World Health Organisation, Geneva, 1995.
12. The NHS and Community Care Act 1990. London: HMSO, 1990.

13. Hine CE, Bachmann MO. What does locality commissioning in Avon offer? Retrospective descriptive evaluation. *Br Med J* 1997;**314**:1246-50.
14. Black DG, Birchall AD, Trimble IMG. Non-fundholding in Nottingham: a vision of the future. *Br Med J* 1994:**309**:930-2.
15. Smith J, Shapiro J. Local call. *Health Serv J* 6 January 1997, pp 26-7.
16. Mays N, Goodwin N, Bevan G, Wyke S. On behalf of the Total Purchasing National Evaluation Team. *Total Purchasing. A Profile of national pilot projects.* London: King's Fund Publishing, 1997.
17. Dixon J, Harrison A. A little local difficulty? *Br Med J* 1997;**314**:216-9.
18. *Continuum of Care. A strategy to improve the interface with primary care.* London: Guy's and St Thomas' Hospital Trust, May 1997.
19. *Designed to Care.* Secretary of State for Scotland. Edinburgh: The Stationery Office Limited, 1997.
20. Audit Commission. *What the doctor ordered. A study of general practitioner fundholders in England and Wales.* London: HMSO, 1996.
21. Petchey R. General practitioner fundholding: weighing the evidence. *Lancet* 1995;**346**:1139-42.
22. Coulter A. Evaluating general practice fundholding in the United Kingdom. *Eur J Public Health* 1995;**5**:223-39.
23. Dixon J, Glennerster H. What do we know about fundholding in general practice? *Br Med J* 1995;**311**:727-30.
24. Dixon J, Dinwoodie M, Hodson D, Dodd S *et al.* Distribution of NHS funds between fundholding and non-fundholding practices. *Br Med J* 1994;**309**:30-4.
25. Glennerster H, Matsaganis M, Owens P, Hancock S. General practitioner fundholding: Wild card or winning hand? In: Robinson R, Le Grand J, Eds. Evaluating the NHS Reforms. London: King's Fund, 1994.
26. Mays N, Dixon J. *Purchaser plurality in UK health care. Is a consensus emerging and is it the right one?* London: King's Fund Publishing, 1996.
27. Robinson JC, Casalino LP. Vertical integration and organizational networks in health care. *Health Affairs* 1996;**15**:7-22.
28. Dale J, Lang H, Roberts JA, Green J, Glucksman E. Cost effectiveness of treating primary care patients in accident and emergency: a comparison between general practitioners, senior house officers, and registrars. *Br Med J* 1966;**312**:1340-44.
29. Pederson LL, Leese B. What will a primary care-led NHS mean for general practitioner workload? The problem of a lack of evidence base. *Br Med J* 1997;**314**:1337-41.
30. Coulter A, Mays N. Deregulating primary care. *Br Med J* 1997;**314**:510-13.
31. Groves T. What the changes mean. *Br Med J* 1997;**314**;436-8.
32. Kendrick T, Hilton S. Broader teamwork in primary care. *Br Med J* 1997;**314**:672-5.
33. Hunter D, Fairfield G. Disease management. *Br Med J* 1997;**315**:50-3.
34. Oxley C, Buchan I. Tracking down Care. *Health Service Journal* 1997;**107**:34–35.
35. Appleby J. *A measure of effectiveness? A critical review of the NHS efficiency index.* Birmingham: National Association of Health Authorities and Trusts, 1996.
36. Kongstvedt PR. Changing provider behaviour in managed care plans. In: Kongstvedt PR, Ed. Essentials of managed health care. Maryland: Aspen Publications, 1995.
37. Ginzberg E, Ostow M. Managed care-a look back and a look ahead. *N Engl J M* 1997;**336**:1018-20.

5 Primary care in an imperfect market

John Roberts

The global move towards health markets, espoused in Britain as the internal market between health professionals but elsewhere involving patients more directly, seems remorseless. If primary care is to influence the direction of market developments, it needs to understand the potentials and the drawbacks to the choices on offer. Nowhere are most of those options concurrently displayed as they are in the United States, from where John Roberts analyses five market systems.

Doctors generally disdain the word "market" when applied to the work they do. A market is an encounter controlled by supply and demand.[1] In most markets there is a purchaser, who pays for the specific goods he will receive and a seller, who has the goods and will provide them to the purchaser.

Medicine is an imperfect market. In health care the purchaser is usually not the consumer, and the goods provided by the seller are difficult to define and often contingent on other aspects of care such as results of tests and treatments.[2] In addition, the medical marketplace does not follow the classic rules of supply and demand. Doctors (to a diminishing extent) set the demand of the care that they will provide, and therefore can artificially increase demand for the goods they supply, highlighted by Roemer's Law: "The supply of beds creates the demand for those beds."[3]

Economic theory also assumes that the buyer-consumer will be knowledgeable about the goods to be purchased and can compare sellers' quality and prices. This is difficult in medicine. Firstly, seller-doctors have until recently controlled all the information about health care. Secondly, consumer-patients tend to avoid using medical services until they need them acutely, and, by then, shopping is virtually impossible. Thirdly, even if payer-insurers or consumer-patients try hard to compare seller-doctors and their products, data are expensive to collect and complex to interpret. Finally, in the UK and in the non-urban and poorer parts of the

US, seller-doctors can set up monopolies or oligopolies in which neither purchasers nor consumer-patients can shop or even easily negotiate services or prices.

Despite these exceptions, it has become increasingly clear over the past 20 years that medicine does behave as a market in many ways. Most obviously, doctors behave according to the rewards they are given. Insurers, whether private or public, can no longer afford unfettered inflation, and have become active buyers willing to invest heavily in comparing costs and quality. In the US purchasers now have more information on the market than the doctors who deliver the services. Consumer-patients, too, respond to market incentives. For example, a small copayment (e.g. $10 at the time of medical service) decreases use of emergency departments by 10-20% .[4,5]

The primary care perspective

So where does primary care fit into the discussion? Primary care, directly accessible 24 hours a day, is usually the patient's first point of contact with the medical system. The primary care physician should be the friend, philosopher, and guide of his or her patients, an advocate and protector and coordinator of appropriate specialist services. He or she should provide long term, continuing, comprehensive care. The primary care physician also acts as a health broker. Within the community, primary care can improve the health of the population through helping to remedy social pathologies, planned health promotion, risk factor screening disease prevention; collection of reliable data on the condition of a community and helping it to decide on priorities for health.[6]

The term "health broker" describes how critical primary care is to any sane medical market. A short history of US medicine shows why. In 1940, 90% of US physicians declared themselves "generalists." When the nation went to war, workers' pay was frozen, so medical insurance quickly became popular as a legal way to make jobs more attractive to workers in short supply. By war's end, most workers were covered by indemnity insurance, which paid doctors for services rendered (fee for service). Not only did this new system reward doctors for testing and treating with little regard to costs, it rewarded patients for seeing the most expensive doctors. These were usually specialists, who dealt with patients whose probability of severe or unusual illness was greater and therefore required greater expenditures. Such unchecked consumerism led to massive cost inflation, the tremendous expansion of speciality medicine, and the near demise of primary care. By the 1980s only about a third of doctors in the US called themselves "generalists."[2]

From consumerism to managed care

The inflation became so burdensome to employers paying for medical insurance that huge companies were being crippled. Chrysler, during the 1980s, was paying more for medical insurance than steel for its cars. One remedy was managed care, which had begun 50 years earlier during the labour movements of the 1930s. In managed care, insurers (usually called health maintenance organisations) pay doctors a prepaid capitation amount for each patient the doctor agrees to care for. In essence, payment is for persons served, not for services delivered. The incentives are the converse of those of fee-for-service medicine, encouraging doctors to spend less and patients to see specialists only rarely.

The rise of capitated care has been slow, but, in the last 20 years, it has come to surpass the fee for service system in primary care. About 55% of Americans are now in some sort of managed care arrangement, and the number may soon jump to 75% as the government embraces managed care as the preferred public insurance mechanism for the poor (through the scheme Medicaid) and elderly (through Medicare).

In general, primary care physicians in managed care behave much like GPs in the UK: they serve as doctors of first resort for nearly all medical problems, and act as gatekeepers for patients' access to specialists. With the rise in managed care has come a parallel rise in the demand for primary care; specialists now have problems finding work in a nation oversupplied by doctors while primary care doctors are still in great (though diminishing) demand.[7] Doctors in training have recognised this new situation and, for the past three years, have chosen the primary care disciplines (family medicine, internal medicine, and paediatrics) rather than speciality training for the first time in several decades.

Five market models

America, as its politicians are fond of boasting, is an experiment, and nowhere is this more true than in medical markets. One cannot generalise about American medicine as one can about UK medicine. Nothing about medical systems is true throughout the country. Los Angeles and its managed care system is both ideologically and geographically a continent away from the Southeast, where fee-for-service medicine still predominates. This somewhat chaotic nation of health care systems illustrates how primary care affects various medical markets, and how they, in turn, affect the practice of primary care. There are at least four models in the US and one other - the single payer - as shown in Table 5.1.

Integrationist

This is the fee-for-service system that many doctors in America still cling to, particularly in much of the eastern seaboard. It remains in place, in an attenuated form, for several reasons. Firstly, it is traditional, so doctors and patients (and even insurers, to some extent) are comfortable with it. Secondly, fee-for service medicine can draw doctors to rural areas, where general practitioner recruitment is often difficult. Thirdly, managed care does best in urban areas, where people can travel short distances to various competing medical centres.

However, for primary care, fee-for-service medicine has generally been detrimental because it rewards oversupply of services and allows patients to bypass the primary care doctor and go directly to the specialist. Obviously, development of community-oriented primary care is impossible in such circumstances.

Outreach

This market model has become popular with academic and other tertiary centres, with their surpluses of specialists. The primary care doctor's surgery remains the centre of clinical activity, and specialists regularly attend sessions there. Such systems have become common in smaller cities, where there are relatively fewer specialists, and among specialities that are extremely overpopulated, such as gastroenterology, cardiology, and orthopaedic surgery. In the Midwestern US, where distances between cities are great, this has become a popular practice. Major medical schools such as those in Chicago and Minneapolis send their faculty members out by aeroplane virtually every day of the week.

For primary care doctors, this system usually works well. A concern is that the outreach system allows more patients with complicated or chronic diseases to bypass their primary care doctors. This trend has been tempered by those who pay for

34

managed care, who believe that speciality care is costlier but rarely better for such patients.

Competitive

This model is common in cities where competition for patients is high, not only between specialists but also between primary care doctors and specialists, and where there are too many doctors. The specialist might tell the asthmatic patient, "Next time you have an attack come and see me directly." Such behaviour undermines the patient's relationship with the primary care doctor, or, when the primary care doctor is meant to be acting as a gatekeeper to each specialist visit, creates outright animosity between the doctors.

One response has been the creation of various types of multi-speciality schemes, where all doctors in a group (including some primary care doctors) share the risk of the costs incurred by the entire practice. If the specialist believes she or he can provide care of equal quality that is cheaper than care offered by the primary care doctor, so much the better, as long as the doctors are working closely together. However, most evidence suggests that specialists are more costly, even when excluding the cost of the sicker patients they see.[8] As specialists learn to become more cost effective this model will probably grow in the US.

Managed Market

This is where America has been heading and is where primary care becomes a true gatekeeper speciality. It is crucial to understand that in the US at present managed care is an extremely competitive and risky marketplace, with more than 1000 insurers trying to sell coverage at lower and lower rates while trying to get doctors to accept more financial risk for patients. The trend now is toward mergers among insurers, which, if carried far enough, will create a landscape that resembles a lot of mini-NHSs.

Two trends are noteworthy. Firstly, the push towards forcing doctors to take on financial risk has caused the demise of the solo primary care practitioner. Doctors are getting together in bigger groups, both formally and informally, in order to promote economies of scale in purchasing supplies and delivering care. Some are adding specialists, moving toward a variation of the outreach and competitive models.[9]

Secondly, very few managed care organisations have convinced the clinical teams to take on all risk. So far, it has been limited

Table 5.1: A model of medical markets, from least to most regulated. Each type of arrangement has advantages and disadvantages, but primary care tends to work best in relatively more regulated markets

	Integrationist	Out-Reach
Description	Traditional self-pay or indeminity insurance in US	Specialists travel to primary care sites to deliver care
Example	Pre-1980 US Generally fee for service More is better	Much of rural US, where services are provided by big urban tertiary care centers
Payers	Public or private Act as funnel for money	Public or private
Advantages:	Minimal administrative costs	Patients not forced to travel far for care, decreasing absenteeism
Disadvantages:	Somewhat at mercy of prividers' charges and behaviour	Insurers actually may seek costs rise, since they will pay specialists' costs but would not pay patients' travel costs to specialty centers
Provider–Doctors	Fee for service	Fee for service or capitation agreements
Advantages:	Doctors control most of spending. Great financial and clinical autonomy	Patients served more conveniently
Disadvantages:	Subject to major changes when payer decides costs much be trimmed. (e.g. current Medicare cuts in US)	Possible threat to primary care if specialists continue to migrate to rural areas
Consumer–Patients	Often pay co-insurance (20% of total charges) or deductibles (first $500 of charges)	Payment types varies
Advantages:	Places some responsibility on patient to keep costs in check	
Disadvantages:	Discriminates against the poor	

Competitive	Managed Market	Single Payer
Specialists compete with primary care doctors for certain diseases	Insurer generally contracts with primary care and other doctors to provide all care in a prepaid scheme	One massive payer, virtually always government, oversees system
Many cities that have not moved to "gatekeeper" or other managed care systems	Health maintenance organizations in most of US	NHS
Public or private	Private > public, but less so	Public
As doctors adopt open competition, costs theoretically should decrease	Can predict costs	Can predict costs
Cost decreases have not been shown due to relatively higher costs of specialists	Little disadvantage as long as patients are satisfied and doctors don't revolt en masse	Political leaders must suffer the pains of public opinion when cost cutting is perceived to damage quality of care
Fee for service or capitation agreements	Usually capitated	Mostly capitated
Specialists gain patients	Primary care doctor usually acts as gatekeeper	Primary care doctor is gatekeeper Community-oriented care is virtually required, since PCPs are assigned patient panels
For primary care: loss of comprehensive care and loss of patients. Specialists may eventually tire of having to provide primary care	Ability to refer may be onerous due to HMO's restriction on specialists. Specialists are completely at mercy of PCPs' referral patterns	Overall limits to spending make quality difficult to maintain If specialists are salaried, they may be overwhelmed by referrals of relatively few patients
Payment types varies	Usually prepared and often with small copayment ($10) at each doctor visit	Prepaid through taxes Usually no co-payment or deductible
Rapid access to specialty care	Patient satisfaction becomes a major determinant of quality care	Primary care, potentially, is practiced at its finest level, with emphasis both on patient and on community
Loss of primary care	Barriers to referrals as described above	Can be difficult for patient to change doctors

mainly to primary care doctors, who get about 10% (typically about $15 per member per month) of the premiums paid to the insurer. Specialists and hospitals have continued to use a mainly fee for service system.

Single payer

The single payer system, as exemplified by the British National Health Service, is used throughout the world, except in the US. Variations on the model are as numerous as the number of nations sponsoring these systems.

The advantages and disadvantages of the single payer system are fairly obvious. Firstly, a nation can set a global budget and decide exactly what it will spend on health care each year. Proponents say that overall medical budgeting is a political issue; critics say this is rationing. Secondly, in systems such as the NHS that rely heavily on primary care, community-oriented primary care becomes the norm, with each doctor responsible for maximising the health of all those patients on a defined, registered list. Thirdly, this list system creates some restriction in choice for patients, especially when, under risk-assuming reforms such as fundholding, there are incentives to under-refer. Fourthly, under global budgeting, some doctors are sure to suffer disproportionately; in the UK, the specialists have to deal with long queues of patients awaiting appointments and elective procedures.

Donald Light has congratulated the UK for its wisdom in creating its system of paying primary care doctors, pointing out that its three-part system of paying capitation, operating costs, and bonuses for targets ensures that patients are neither overtreated (as in the US fee for service system) or undertreated (a potential risk of the for-profit managed care schemes in the US).[10] The single payer system does not, however, foster experimentation and entrepreneurship; if a better idea comes along it has to be implemented through regional or national bureaucracies.

Conclusions

The marketplace cannot solve the problems of medicine, nor eradicate the tensions between primary care and specialist doctors. Nor can an imperfect model ensure highest quality medicine at the lowest costs.

But in considering primary care medicine and the marketplace, it may be helpful to turn to a failed reform of the American system, that of President Clinton's in the early 1990s. His task force, while realising that an imperfect market can never be made truly perfect, did list five criteria for an optimal medical market (Box 5.1).

Box 5.1

1 Universal medical insurance coverage.
2 Costs that are affordable to society and to patients.
3 Comprehensive medical benefits.
4 Freedom of patients to choose their own doctors.
5 Public accountability, both in cost and in quality of care.

Unfortunately, these five statements are probably mutually exclusive in practice. But they remain a goal for all of us to consider as we continue to reform our own medical marketplaces.

1 Stoline AM, Weiner JP. *The New Medical Marketplace: A Physician's Guide to the Health Care System in the 1990s*. Baltimore: The Johns Hopkins Press, 1993.
2 Light DW. Health care systems and their financing. In: Walton J, Barondess JA, Lock S, Eds. *The Oxford Medical Companion*. Oxford: Oxford University Press, 1994.
3 Feldstein P. *Health Care Economics*, 2nd ed. New York: John Wiley and Sons, 1994.
4 O'Grady KF, Maning WG, Newhouse JP, Borrk RH. The impact of cost sharing on emergency department use. *N Engl J Med* 1985;313:484-90.
5 Selby JV, Fireman BH, Swain BE. Effect of a copayment on use of the ED in an HMO. *N Engl J Med* 1996;334:635-41.
6 Fry J, Light D, Rodnick J, Orton P. *Reviving Primary Care: A US-UK Comparison*. Oxford: Radcliffe Medical Press, 1995.
7 Miller RS, Jonas HS, Whitcomb ME. The initial employment status of physicians completing training in 1994. *JAMA* 1996;275:708-12.
8 Greenfield S, Nelson EC, Zubkoff M, Manning W, Rogers W, Kravitz RL, *et al.* Variations in resource utilization among medical specialties and systems of care: results from the medical outcomes study. *JAMA* 1992;267:1624-30.
9 Medical leadership Council. *Report from the Frontier, 1997*. Washington: The Advisory Board, 1997.
10 Light DW. Primary medical care: more choice, less cost. *Med Care* 1996;34:985-6.

6 Patient priorities

Rabbi Julia Neuberger

The recent NHS reforms have been driven by political pressures and, to an extent, professional needs. Patients have been expressing their views but it is difficult to see evidence of their effect on policy. Yet now, as the health service comes under pressure, is an important time for primary care to refocus on patients' priorities.

In this chapter Julia Neuberger looks at one recent change - the revolution in out of hours care - as an example of the current state of patient influence. As the chapter develops, Neuberger explores the roles of primary care practitioners as providers of patient friendly services, conduits towards alternative medicine, and as advocates for patients who need to use hospital and social services.

Designing services: whose agenda?

How to run a twenty-four hour system of general practice has been a bone of contention between general practitioners and the public in recent years.[1][2] Doctors are loath to continue doing their own on call work at nights and weekends.[3][4] Patients, however, undoubtedly prefer to see their own doctor or a general practitioner from their own practice[5][6] where the service may be better[7], rather than a doctor from an agency that provides the on-call service.[8][9]

This is the nub of the difference in perception between doctors and patients (and to some extent between health care professionals and the general public) about the quality of service they would like to see, and that difference in perception is one which needs to be taken seriously. When asked, patients express a wish to be involved in planning services and their delivery[10][11] and practices find this process worthwhile.[11][12] And yet, radical changes in out of hours services have occurred without overt consultation with patients.

The starting point

Our general practitioner service in particular, and our primary care services in general, are the jewel in the NHS crown for much of the British public.[13] There is no doubt that the vast majority of the population regards the general practitioner as their first port of call for healthcare, and as the health professional they trust (on the whole, despite concerns about fundholding) to give them advice and treatment. They recognise the need for a guide through the maze of services that make up our increasingly complex health service.

A simple first priority for most patients is getting really good advice from their primary health care providers. That advice includes such details as what the best treatment for a particular condition might be, and what the downside to it might be[14]; who or where would provide that treatment and where the highest success rates are to be found. Indeed, there is some irritation amongst the general public at the lack of openness on the part of the profession about success rates from procedures, although some evaluations are available.[15]

Anecdotally, people point out that doctors always know where, and to whom, they would rather go to be treated for particular conditions, and where they would send their family - and they cannot see why that kind of information should not be directly available to them. They access this knowledge indirectly through the general practitioners' choice of referral, but objective evidence on which to judge specific hospitals, units and consultants is still not available.

It also has to be recognised that the patients' definition of success may not be the same as the health care professionals', and that increasingly the public expects to get its definition of quality and benefit recognised. The emphasis on biomedical outcomes used by health care professionals or health economists has to be tempered with a recognition of patients' definitions of outcome.

This applies to preferences concerning general practices themselves. While partnerships get bigger and teams more complex, patients express greater satisfaction with smaller practices[16] which are not involved in training[17] and run personal registered lists.[18] Patients appear to be valuing different characteristics to those given greatest priority by general practitioners and this will inevitably lead to tensions.

Patients want to know what the choices are for people with various forms of chronic conditions and where the best alleviation can be found. These days they expect to have access to a full primary health care team[19 20] and to be advised to use alternative forms of health care if they seem valuable – notably osteopathy and chiropractic, but also aromatherapy (for some end-stage cancer patients and for women who have chronic severe mental illness) and acupuncture (for intractable pain). That advice is now seen as part of the armoury for living with illness and chronic conditions, and therefore a part of health care advice that people expect from the primary health care team.

Accessibility

High priority is put on out of hours services by the general public. That applies to the on call service, and to the sense of general lack of availability of primary health care services over public holidays. In personal discussions, there is an increasingly strong feeling that primary health care services should be available, at least in part, on some of those holidays, so that the public is not kept away from those services for up to four days over, say, Christmas and Easter.

That is particularly true for certain groups of patients and their families. If primary care is to mean anything to much of the population, it has to be based on the notion that people live with families, partners or carers, and that part of the role of the primary care team is to care for the rest of the family. So, for instance, the very fact that services are not available for four days over some public holidays makes many of those who live with severely mentally ill people angry, and renders them helpless. There is a strong feeling that primary care services for certain groups, notably the mentally ill and the elderly, should be better in general and more widely available in terms of hours of service.

Extending the concept of primary care

Patients often report that they express their views to their general practitioners and primary health care teams but are not listened to. They feel that their priorities are different from those of the practice team, and that there should be more fundamental questioning of whom the service is for, and how it can be provided more in accord with patient needs.

Patients want to be listened to [10-12], both about their demands for health care, and in general. The growth of counselling being available in primary care is certain evidence of the need for listening of professional quality.[21] The problem for many patients is the very variable quality of counselling services offered, from the highly professional thoroughly trained, to those who have attended a short course. The British Association for Counselling's register and gradual licensing of counsellors is much to be welcomed, but it needs urgent implementation. The concerns of members of the public about quality of counselling and the amount of counselling they are offered in primary health care need to be addressed.

Patients also want a wider range of services to be easily available, be it physiotherapy (always much in demand and something that could, in the larger practices, be made available), podiatry, osteopathy or consultant sessions for common conditions that require referral. But it is not only health care services that the public wishes to see. As primary care expands its range of interests and skills, it becomes more essential that we should see primary care centres as one-stop shops for those services which are determinants of health. These include housing, and some social services in addition to the current system of health care.

This is not to suggest that all housing offices for a local area should be made available at health centres (though that might not be too bad a development), but that those housing services targeted at elderly people, people with enduring mental illness or learning difficulties, could receive specialist housing advice from representatives of local authorities or housing associations based within the health centres.

That is equally true of advice on welfare benefits, and there is good reason to think of Citizens' Advice Bureaux operating from within health centres along with social services, especially those which are targeted at people with chronic poor health. Indeed, it is extraordinary that, in our well-developed primary health care system in the UK, so little development of joint premises for health and other services has taken place. Since primary care is going to be increasingly the focus of services, and the gateway to them, it is essential that other services are to be found under the same roof. Only that way can a primary health care worker be certain that adequate social services are being provided for a very dependent patient.

Indeed, it could be argued that general practitioners and other primary health care workers, such as district nurses, should be orchestrating the services that enable people who are severely handicapped, for whatever reason, to stay in their own homes. That is particularly important for the elderly, and the role of the primary health care team in ensuring elderly people stay in their own homes as long as possible, properly supported, is clearly one which needs further development. Primary health care teams can orchestrate services for elderly and other patients, but only if their access to other service providers is good, one reason at least why social services and housing should be found in health centres.

The practice team members as advocates

The public looks to health professionals, and particularly general practitioners, to help them to access services. However, the reality is that the advocacy role - so often claimed by primary health care professionals - needs developing if assisting access to services is to become a major role.

Just as mental health care requires an integrated approach, services for the elderly raise issues of access, advocacy and coordination. The range of models from general practitioner or nurse managed services, to low key units offering outreach of specialist care from the acute section (as has been so successfully piloted by Lambeth Community NHS Trust), requires active management. As the movement of services out of hospitals continues, the role of the primary health care team in delivering less acute in patient services will need to be explored, including a possible return to provision of local cottage hospitals. Such a choice may well prove to be a valuable answer for elderly people and their families.

Meanwhile, the public is worried by some questions over ownership of nursing homes by general practitioners - a move that creates a conflict of interest and undermines the doctors' advocacy role. In the light of more general anxieties about standards in nursing homes, it could be argued that the primary health care team could act as an impartial unofficial inspection team of these and other community based institutions, since their interest must be the patients' welfare, rather than the profit motive of the owner.

Lastly, there is a perceived need for general practitioners and primary health care workers to act as advocates of particular groups of patients. Where the patient group is genuinely inarticulate and has no-one else to stand up for them, health professionals may play a vital role - a role that is limited at present.

There is always a danger when health professionals take on the mantle of the patient's advocate or friend; professional interests and concerns can differ from personal ones, and some distance needs to be maintained. Nevertheless, the public expects the primary health care team to orchestrate services, advise, inspect services, and educate.

Conclusions

In this chapter I have reflected on the conflict between the priorities that patients, the consumers of the health service, express and the aspirations of general practitioners and their teams. To an extent this can be overcome by increased communication and patient participation. However, primary care services could do much more to meet patients' needs through offering extended advocacy. Vulnerable and other groups will increasingly look to primary care teams to lead community action on housing and benefits, as well as ensuring equal access to high quality health and social care.

1. O'Dowd T, Sinclair H. Open all hours: night visits in general practice. *Br Med J* 1994;**308**:1386.
2. Heath I. General practice at night. *Br Med J* 1995;**311**:466.
3. Lattimer V, Smith H, Hungin P, Glasper A, George S. Future provision of out of hours primary medical care: a survey with two general practitioner research networks. *Br Med J* 1996;**312**:352-6.
4. Salisbury C. Evaluation of a general practice out of hours cooperative: a questionnaire survey of general practitioners. *Br Med J* 1997;**314**:1598-9.
5. Salisbury C. Postal survey of patients' satisfaction with a general practice out of hours cooperative. *Br Med J* 1997;**314**:1594-8.
6. McKinley R, Cragg D, Hastings A, French D, Manku-Scott T, Campbell S, et al. Comparison of out of hours care provided by patients' own general practitioners and comercial deputising services: a randomised controlled trial. II: The outcome of care. *Br Med J* 1997;**314**:190-3.
7. Crogg D, McKinley R, Roland M, Campbell S, Van F, Hastings A, et al. Comparison of out of hours care provided by patients' own general practitioners and commercial deputising services: a randomised controlled trial. I: The process of care. *Br Med J* 1997;**314**:187-9.
8. Salisbury C. Observational study of a general practice out of hours cooperative: measures of activity. *Br Med J* 1997;**314**:182-6.
9. Jessopp L, Beck I, Hollins L, Shipman C, Reynolds M, Dale J. Changing the pattern out of hours: a survey of general practice cooperatives. *Br Med J* 1997;**314**:199-200.
10. Maeseneer J. Priority setting in general practice at the local level: from patient participation to community orientation? *Eur J Gen Pract* 1996;**2**:3-4.
11. Pringle M, Wallis H, Fairbairn S. Involving practice staff and patients in determining standards and priorities in primary care. *Eur J Gen Pract* 1996;**2**:5-8.
12. Hearnshaw H, Baker R, Cooper A, Eccles M, Soper J. The costs and benefits of asking patients their opinions about general practice. *Family Practice* 1996;**13**:52-8.
13. Calnan M, Katsouyiannopoulos V, Ovcharov V, Prokhorskas R, Ramic H, Williams S. Major determinants of consumer satisfaction with primary care in different health systems. *Family Practice* 1994;**11**:468-78.

14. Britten N. Patients' demands for prescriptions in primary care. *Br Med J* 1995;**310**:1084-5.
15. Brown J, Smith R, Cantor T, Chesover D, Yearsley R. General practitioners as providers of minor surgery - a success story? *British Journal of General Practice* 1997;**47**:205-10.
16. Campbell J. The reported availability of general practitioners and the influence of practice list size. *British Journal of General Practice* 1996;**46**:465-8.
17. Baker R, Streatfield J. What type of general practice do patients prefer? Exploration of practice characteristics influencing patient satisfaction. *British Journal of General Practice* 1995;**45**:654-9.
18. Baker R. Characteristics of practices, general practitioners and patients related to levels of patients' satisfaction with consultations. *British Journal of General Practice* 1996;**46**:601-5.
19. Heath I. Skill Mix in primary care. *Br Med J* 1994;**308**:993-4.
20. Kendrick D. Role of the primary health care team in preventing accidents to children. *British Journal of General Practice* 1994;**44**:372-5.
21. Spiers R, Jewell J. One counsellor; two practices: report of a pilot scheme in Cambridgeshire. *British Journal of General Practice* 1995;**45**:31-3.

7 Evidence and general practice care

Chris Van Weel

The objective of general practice is to provide personal, ongoing care for patients in their social and family context. As part of its commitment to such care, general practice should reflect established best practice in medicine in a framework of prevailing ethical and moral values. This is the basis of the Hippocratic oath and is where the core values of the discipline of general practice originated.

This chapter examines the importance of evidence based medicine for general practice. It focuses less on the application of available evidence in daily practice, but more on the contribution of evidence for the specific mission of general practice in health care. This analysis will be constructed around a case history that allows consideration of the sort of evidence that is needed to fulfil that mission.

A case history

Sylvia Evans is a 61 year old retired school teacher. For four years she has been treated for non-insulin dependent diabetes mellitus but she has achieved less than satisfactory metabolic control. Despite concerted efforts, her random blood glucose readings vary between 9.5–11.8 mmol/l. Dietary advice has not resulted in a significant loss of weight and her body mass index remains at 30.4. Tolbutamide, and later glibenclamide, resulted in feelings of depression without signs of hypoglycaemia and these drugs had to be discontinued. Insulin therapy provoked restlessness and anxiety - again without evidence that these symptoms were caused by low blood glucose.

Mrs. Evans lives with her husband who is eight years older and severely handicapped by a combination of Parkinsonism and mild dementia. The couple live independently and Mrs. Evans spends virtually all her time caring for her husband. All other things in life come second to this - including concerns for her diabetes mellitus.

47

One of the most significant innovations in general practice in recent years has been the advent of protocols, guidelines and standards[1]: recommendations for routine general practice treatment and care, usually based on the best available scientific data. This evidence base can be seen, for example, in the comprehensive approach of the Dutch College of General Practitioners for developing and implementing standard guidelines for common health problems in primary care.[1,2] Behind each proposed guideline lies a systematic review of the available literature on that subject. A group of experts from primary care weigh and discuss this evidence, and prepare guidelines for the most important clinical decisions general practitioners have to make for that health problem. Areas where evidence is weak, or not available, are clarified, and then the available evidence is used to create standards of current best practice. Each standard is published with its supporting evidence[2], a process undertaken for diabetes mellitus.[3] The Dutch recommendations for diabetes mellitus do not differ significantly from the British guidelines.[4]

The case of Sylvia Evans presents her general practitioner with a number of challenges.

Sylvia Evans' doctor, as a conscientious general practitioner, reviews the available guidelines and examines the most important papers in the scientific literature. This review, necessarily selectively reported here for the purposes of illustrating the argument, confirms the familiar biomedical approach to care.

The doctor finds a long term descriptive study published in 1995 which pointed to the poor prognosis and high frequency of cardiovascular morbidity and mortality among patients with non insulin dependent diabetes mellitus (NIDDM).[5] This study was undertaken on a cohort of patients from general practice, and the findings could be generalised to patients like Mrs Evans. This study provides support for regarding Sylvia Evans, with her poor control, as at increased risk of cardiovascular complications.

The doctor establishes that obesity, abnormalities of lipid metabolism and hyperglycaemia are common pathways of atherogenesis[6], and this points to the potential of prevention and intervention. In this respect NIDDM is different from chronic arthritis, irritable bowel syndrome or migraine, where conceptual understanding is poor or conflicting, and can offer only ambiguous guidance. Recent publications demonstrate the efficacy of metabolic control in NIDDM[7,8], consistent lowering of blood glucose being accompanied by a more favourable prognosis.

The general practitioner accepts that these findings are valid for patients like Mrs Evans. Lowering her blood glucose levels can, therefore, be seen as an evidence-based treatment objective - a statement not only based on the significance of the p values or confidence intervals of the intervention studies, but one that is also consistent with theoretical concepts about diabetes.

The limitations of the evidence based approach

In the case of Mrs Evans this is not the end of the trail. The prognosis of poorly controlled NIDDM is clearly established, as is the extent to which strict metabolic control can improve this prognosis. However, the drugs used in the intervention studies had already been prescribed and had resulted in perceived adverse effects. Mrs Evans's general practitioner might seek an alternative drug, and could accompany her prescription with counselling on the true nature of the side effects which Sylvia Evans experienced.

Both of these additional interventions interfere, however, with the evidence basis for action - at least in theory. The intervention studies were conducted using the very drugs that caused the adverse effects, but not with any available alternatives. Each clinical study can offer results which apply only in the circumstances in which the research was conducted, thus the assumption of comparable benefits from a related but not studied drug requires a clinical judgement based on circumstantial evidence.

Secondly, and more intriguing, is the contextual application of an intervention that has gained the evidence-based trademark. Good general practice care will require education, information, counselling, and support, in addition to the intervention. But this approach to care is an essential deviation from the way drugs are prescribed in clinical trials that provide evidence of effectiveness. The therapeutic transfer that accompanies prescribing in real life cannot be controlled for in a randomised controlled trial. For general practitioners, therefore, there is seldom proof of any intervention's effectiveness under real life circumstances unless observational studies have been conducted.

Asking a different question

A different, but just as important, set of questions about Mrs Evans's care concern the effects of tight metabolic control on this woman's functional status, its interference with her ability to care for her husband, and how this would affect the health status of Mr Evans and the wellbeing of the couple. Mrs Evans's main concern is her ability to continue caring for her husband; the effect of interventions on this aspect of her life must be considered. Clinical trials should, but seldom do, report on patient as well as disease outcomes, such as quality of life, perceived health, and functional status.

Mrs Evans's general practitioner therefore looks for studies that have included such patient oriented measures in NIDDM. Though tight supervision of diabetes does wonders for the patients' blood glucose, its consequences for the patients' functional status might at least be ambivalent or contradictory.[9]

Evidence and the mission of general practice

For Sylvia Evans the prime outcome of care for her diabetes is sufficient wellbeing to allow her to care for her husband, while for many doctors and in most studies the prime outcome is effect on clinical disease progression. This discrepancy shows that evidence should relate to patients' expectations of outcome as well as doctors', and that studies should be designed to address both agendas.

Evidence based medicine is the methodology of finding watertight scientific answers to questions that follow from patient care[10] while the mission statement of general practice is to formulate objectives for patient care in their sociocultural context. Patients' perspectives and priorities (see Chapter 6)[9] and the whole contextual setting of care (available time and resources)[11] are vital parts of the primary care ethos which remain unexplored in randomised controlled trials.

Where there is good quality evidence available, it can guide the general practitioner or further develop the discipline[3] - provided the question answered is a suitable one. This underlines the need for general practice based evidence, as well as general practice based guidelines and standards. And it highlights the need for all well-founded evidence to be made available. The justification for masterly inactivity (or watchful waiting), that irrefutably valuable part of general practice, rests largely on numerous reports of interventions which have no effect - and this is despite the continuing bias towards publishing positive findings. If negative findings are not made available, evidence will inevitably emphasise the case for rather than against intervening.

As the case study shows, when available evidence is irrelevant to the question being addressed by the clinician and the patient, the reality is that there is no evidence. Under these circumstances general practitioners have to do what they have always done - exercise their professional judgement and guide the patient towards management strategies that offer, in their informed opinion, the best possible benefit with the least probability of harm. Evidence based clinical practice under these conditions can be seen, not so much as the application of research findings, but as an affirmation of the core values of general practice (see Chapter 1).

Conclusions

Evidence based medicine has an important place in general practice, as it can make a powerful contribution to safe, effective, and efficient care for patients. Whether it will succeed in informing the decisions made with real patients in everyday consultations will depend crucially on whether it offers enough information that is specific to the context of primary care.

Research must embrace the core values of primary care and assess the interventions and outcomes relevant to consultations, and the professional framework of general practice's core values must include the application of evidence whenever relevant. For this to happen, research must focus on common health problems rather than exciting but rare conditions, and must assess the role of interventions other than pharmacological ones.

If this can be achieved, evidence based medicine will serve the ulterior motive of medical care: that it be personal, reasonable, humane, equal, fair, and accountable, and not just a cookbook formula based on the strength of a p value in the answer to a different question.

1. Grol R. Development of guidelines for general practice care. *Br J Gen Pract* 1993; 43: 146-151.
2. Thomas S, Geijer RMM, van der Laan JR, Wiersma Tj. NHG Standaarden voor de huisarts II. Utrecht, wetenschappelijke uitgeverij Bunge, 1996.
3. Cromme PVM, Mulder JD, Rutten GEHM, Zuidweg J, Thomas S. NHG Standaard diabetes mellitus type II. *Huisarts Wet* 1989; 32: 15-18.
4. Clinical Standards Advisory Group. *Standards of clinical care for people with diabetes.* London:HMSO, 1989.
5. de Grauw WJC, van de Lisdonk EH, van den Hoogen HJM, van Weel C. Cardiovascular morbidity and mortality in type-2 diabetic patients: a 22-year historic cohort study in Dutch general practice. *Diabetic Med* 1995; 12: 117-122.
6. Reaven GM. Role of insulin resistance in human disease. *Diabetes* 1988; 37: 1595-1607.

7. Klein R, Klein BEK, Moss SE. Relation of glycaemic control to diabetes microvascular complications in diabetes mellitus. *Ann Intern Med* 1996; **124:** 90-96.

8. Savage PJ Cardiovascular complications of diabetes mellitus: what we know and what we need to know about their prevention. *Ann Intern Med* 1996; **124:** 123-126.

9. de Grauw WJC, van de Lisdonk EH, van Gerwen WHEM, Behr R, van den Hoogen HJM, van Weel C. Functional health status in patients with type-II diabetes in Dutch general practice. Submitted.

10. Sackett DL, Rosenburg WMC, Gray JAM, Haynes RB, Richardson WS. Evidence based medicine: what it is and what it isn't. *Br Med J* 1996; **312:** 71-2.

11. Ridsdale L. *Evidence-based general practice - a critical reader.* London: WB Saunders, 1995.

8 From education and training to professional development

Jacky Hayden

Earlier chapters in this book have identified changes in the way that health care is delivered. They have also identified key characteristics of primary care in the United Kingdom that need to be preserved if we are to retain a service that is acceptable to patients and is cost effective.

In order to consider the part that education might play in delivering effective primary care, it is important to try to determine what the health needs of local populations are likely to be. It is also important to consider how technology and the nature of the workforce may alter, so that educational programmes facilitate the development of a cohort of health care workers who are equipped to work in the new health service.

Charles Handy has already observed that the only predictable element when looking towards the future is that there will be change.[1] Some of the characteristics of future populations are predictable: for example, the population will be older, with an ageing cohort of carers looking after them. At the same time, the size of the tax paying group will diminish in relative terms, and technological developments are likely to encourage shorter stays in secondary care and an increasing ability to undertake more care in the community.

Recent government policy in the UK[2,3] demands that the future provision of most health care will be as near to the patient as possible and will be offered by a team of appropriately trained individuals, similar to today's health care teams working in general medical practice. What is not yet clear is the balance between primary care and self care or support groups.[4]

The General Medical Council's report *Tomorrow's Doctors*[5] has already identified the need for medical students to graduate with a

53

range of skills that will be important to them as doctors of the future. These skills include team working, basing decisions on evidence, and the ability to communicate. Now *The New Doctor*[6] highlights the importance of the learning environment in developing professional values, a concept that is not new to general practice trainers[7] and one that has recently been identified as crucial to the profession of medicine.[4,8]

This chapter considers how education for primary care might alter in response to central policy[2,3,9] and how education might shape the future by contributing to the development of a new kind of workforce.

Education for working in primary care

The current system of education for all health care groups needs to be reviewed. If we expect a range of professionals to work together to deliver care for individual patients and groups of patients there needs to be greater understanding of roles between and within the professions. All health professionals will need programmes of education that are broadly compatible; where possible learning skills that are generic to more than one group might take place in a multiprofessional setting.

More clinical placements in which students from a range of health care backgrounds work together with effective health care teams may break down the barriers which seem to exist at qualification. As the health service recognises the importance of partnerships of care between the patient, their family, and the health care workers, communicating effectively with patients and groups of patients will become more important. With the growing need for evidence based care, sharing of information systems might even encourage a range of health professions to learn critical evaluation together.

Basic education

Changes have already been made to the undergraduate medical curriculum and the basic nursing curriculum. There is greater emphasis on professional skills and values rather than knowledge and many universities are using a problem based approach to learning. The pre-existing structure of assessment of knowledge at the end of basic training seems no longer appropriate; competitive examinations which are peer referenced tend to produce individuals who are themselves competitive rather than collaborative.

Assessment of knowledge will need to be augmented by assessment of skills such as problem solving, communication, team working, management, and critical evaluation skills, such as the ability to interpret research studies.

Traditionally much of the basic education for health care workers, especially medical students, has taken place in teaching hospitals. This setting risks focusing the curriculum too narrowly on a small spectrum of diseases. Universities are increasingly using primary care as a location for clinical experience for medical and non-medical students. There is, however, little coordination between medical and non-medical teachers and supervisors in terms of setting standards for practices and shifting or pooling resources.

The early years in the health service

Experience in the period of training or working immediately after qualification may colour a young person's view of the NHS. Responsibility without confidence or competence often leads to distress and disillusionment. The General Medical Council is now explicit about the standards it expects in training for pre-registration house officers[6]. The amendment to the medical act allows more opportunity for pre-registration experience in general practice. There is still, however, some confusion about how the year could best be used to encourage young doctors to gain a wider perspective of the health service, develop skills in working with other health care workers, and acquire confidence in their clinical and managerial skills.

The pre-registration year seems an ideal time for doctors to experience primary care. The longitudinal perspective of patients' lives, one of the characteristics of working in general practice, would allow them to think about the impact of illness on the family and of the environment on health. It should also allow them to observe how a team of professionals provides care and support to individuals and groups of patients and how the team interfaces with social care.

Wherever the learning takes place, it is important that appropriate professional values in relation to other members of the health care team are established. Health care teams of the future will need individuals who are prepared to work with other professions, respecting different perspectives and priorities. It is essential that

55

the new doctor or recently qualified nurse is exposed to role models who have a strong respect for their own professional values and a high regard for other health professionals.

Specific training for general practice

The nature and scope of general practice has changed immensely since the introduction of vocational training. The supplementary Report on General Practice[10] has proposed further changes in the system of training for general practice. Currently, two thirds of the training continues to take place in hospital practice. Although it is possible to slant the learning towards general practice for senior house officers on formal training schemes, this is only about half of all doctors training for general practice. The other half will submit their experience retrospectively. This effectively means that their specific training for general practice is limited to twelve months.

The future looks brighter, at least for the medical profession. *Delivering the Future*[3] specifically addressed the need for a more even balance between learning in general practice and hospital. Now that the specialist registrar grade has completed transition, postgraduate deans will need to work with their directors of postgraduate general practice education to consider how programmes of education for general practice can be developed within existing resources. It should be possible to create programmes that specifically meet the needs of prospective general practitioners.

These programmes could allow the General Practice Registrar more time working in outpatients, including those of greater relevance to general practice, such as dermatology, ENT and ophthalmology. If we are to expect these doctors to take a lead in developing practice for the next century we also need to set aside time in their curriculum for them to learn the skills necessary to work effectively in a practice team and to provide the leadership which will be required if the practice is to respond to the changing demands of the health service. Although the minimum time needed to train for general practice is three years, it should be possible to create some rotations that include an additional period in practice. There have already been some pilots testing this idea.

Although there are moves towards greater preparation for nursing in the community, more attention is needed to developing the skills necessary to work as a practice nurse and nurse practitioner in primary care. As nurse education has moved to universities, the opportunities for higher degrees have increased. However, it is essential that those nurses who have chosen a career in primary care are offered opportunities to learn skills appropriate to their future work patterns.

Professions allied to medicine have traditionally trained in secondary care, where specialisation has been encouraged. If more of their work is likely to be in primary care we need to consider how their training might embrace a more generalist approach.

Developing practice teams

Perhaps the greatest opportunity for primary care is the review of continuing professional development, chaired by the Chief Medical Officer. Having worked with separate systems of accreditation of education there is now an opportunity for all professions within primary care to establish a mechanism that will encourage practice and professional development to meet the needs of patients.

One of the issues facing primary care is whether its doctors should be self regulating or subject to external review. The General Medical Services Committee has published a framework for reaccreditation of general practitioners[11] and the Royal College of General Practitioners has developed a tool for assessing a practitioner for Fellowship of the College[12].

The professions working within primary care need to consider how they will jointly assure the public that they are maintaining high quality standards of care. Reaccreditation of individuals within the team may be one solution; a stronger solution might be for each practice to identify its own goals and work systematically towards achieving them. The goals will have to be set according to the needs of the population served, the practice and the individuals working in it, and local and national priorities. Progress towards the goals should be monitored using audit. Co-ordinating the professions within the practice will need leadership and sensitivity.

Once a practice has clear, documented goals, it will be able to audit progress towards them and to identify the individual development needs for each member of the health care team. These individual professional development plans should include the needs of the individual, the practice development needs, and local priorities (Figure 8.1). The professional development plans could be documented through a portfolio, which might be reviewed with a mentor[13].

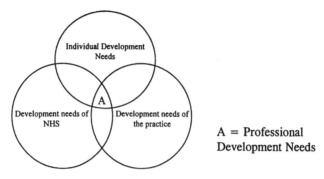

A = Professional
Development Needs

Figure 8.1 Diagram to show professional development needs

Shaping the future

Current changes within the health service have created opportunities to consider how education might influence the future shape of the workforce. With the demise of the Regional Health Authorities, Education and Training Consortia have been established. These consortia bring together health authorities, trusts, general practice, social services, and the voluntary sector. The consortia are coordinated by the Regional Education and Development Group, which also includes the postgraduate deans, directors of postgraduate general practice education, and regional directors.

There is, therefore, an opportunity for each region to consider how it will prepare future and existing generations for work in primary care. One of the greatest barriers that we all face in achieving effective health care is professional rivalry and tribalism. The NHS changes provide an opportunity for all professions in primary care to review what sort of practice we need for our patients and how best to provide it. The next generation should learn in an environment which values the autonomy of patients, the contribution of other professions, the maintenance of clinical knowledge and skills and effective management systems.

1. Handy C *The Age of Unreason*. Second ed. London: Business Books Limited, 1991.
2. Department of Health. *Choice and Opportunity*. London: The Stationery Office, 1996.
3. Department of Health. *Primary Care: Delivering the Future* London: The Stationery Office, 1996.
4. Irvine D. The performance of doctors. 1: Professionalism and self regulation in a changing world. *Br Med J* 1997; **314** 1540-1542.
5. General Medical Council. *Tomorrow's Doctors: Recommendations on undergraduate medical education.*London: GMC, 1993.

6. General Medical Council. *The new doctor.* London: GMC. 1997.
7. Marinker M. *Medical education and human values. J R Coll Gen Prac* 1974; **24** 445-462.
8. Calman K. *The profession of medicine. Br Med J* 1994; **309**: 1140-1143.
9. Department of Health. *The National Health Service - A Service with Ambitions.* London: The Stationery Office, 1996.
10. NHS Executive. *Hospital Doctors: Training for the Future. Supplementary Reports by The Working Groups Commissioned to Consider the Implications for General Medical Practice, Overseas Doctors and Academic and Research Medicine.* 1995.
11. GMSC Education and Audit Subcommittee. *Interim report on individual reaccreditation.* General Medical Services Committee, Annual Report, 1996, 60-66.
12. Royal College of General Practitioners. *Fellowship by Assessment. Occasional Paper 50.* London: RCGP, 1990.
13. Royal College of General Practitioners. *Portfolio-based Learning in General Practice. Occasional Paper 63.* Exeter: RCGP, 1993

9 Primary care, health, and the good society

Dr Iona Heath

To identify and urge the good and achievable society may well be a minority effort, but better that effort than none at all.[1]

The election result of May 1st 1997 brought a profound change of political context for health care services in the United Kingdom. As he took office as Prime Minister, Tony Blair promised a National Health Service rebuilt as the pride of the nation. We seem once again to have a government committed to building a more cohesive and equitable society and affirming the position of the National Health Service as a central part of that society. This chapter examines the role of primary health care, in its components which include general practice, primary care, public health, community action, and social policy, in a good society – and the complementary relationship between them.

There is such a thing as society

Throughout most of the 1970s and 1980s the NHS remained explicitly committed to providing a universal, accessible, and equitable service[2] but was expected to do so within a society which, apparently abhorring equity, was undergoing a rapid process of socioeconomic polarisation. Those working in the frontline of the health service felt frighteningly exposed to the adverse health consequences of these rapid social changes.[3] The challenge now is to reverse these processes through rebuilding the cohesive social structures which generate and promote health in its widest sense.[4] Recognition that this task goes way beyond the NHS has been signalled by the appointment of a minister of public health with an intersectoral brief.

However, the building of the necessary links between health services and other social agencies is impaired by the persistent blurring of the crucial distinction between general practice and primary health care. General practice is an essential component of primary health care, but it is only a small part of the totality. Yet the terms general practice and primary care are often used as if they were almost synonymous, with the implication that general medical practitioners need only to cede some of their traditional control to the other health care disciplines with whom they now work in "primary health care teams" for general practice to become primary care. This confusion is destructive of both entities in ways which appear to have been little recognised.

Illness, disease and health

The principal focus of general practice must be illness, that of primary care should be health. Illness is an often insidious feeling that all is not well with one's body or mind.[5] It is made up of symptoms and is entirely subjective. It is necessarily an intensely individual and thereby lonely experience. It carries an implicit fear that the feeling may be the first harbinger of decay and death, yet the symptoms of illness can be caused by both disease and unhappiness.

Disease, in contrast, is objective and is the unit of the taxonomy by which medical science has attempted to make sense of the undifferentiated mass of subjective human suffering. To caricature, illness is what patients have on the way to the doctor, disease is what they have on the way home. Illness is objectified as disease in the clinical encounter and in that way the fear which is implicit in illness becomes explicit. Once the illness is named as a disease, a rough prognosis can be estimated. Fellow sufferers offer solidarity and help to reduce the loneliness of disease.

In complete contrast, health is essentially positive. It is associated with a feeling of wellbeing with dimensions that are both individual and social. The health of individuals has much to do with how society organises itself in terms of equity, opportunity, cohesion, environment, and culture. Health has very little to do with medicine or indeed with any of the health care disciplines.

To summarise, disease is the stuff of scientific medicine, health is mostly a product of society, and illness is what brings patients to doctors and is therefore the special province of general practice.

The strengths of primary care

The rich industrialised countries have much to learn from the poorer countries of the developing world about the potential of primary care as described and promoted by the World Health

Organisation.[6] Such primary care is undertaken by local communities for local communities, making use of local knowledge and expertise. Primary care is predominantly concerned with the socioeconomic and environmental determinants of health and works to empower local communities to seek to increase their control of these determinants. In this way primary care resists the medicalisation of health. The pretence that general practice is primary care works in the opposite direction.

The strengths of general practice are quite different. General practice provides personal care focused on the individual patient, albeit in the context of their family and community. The particular expertise of the clinical generalist is in acting as both a guardian and an interpreter at the interface between illness and disease.[7] This involves special skills which include being prepared to tolerate uncertainty, and using time as both a diagnostic and a therapeutic tool.

General practice offers continuity and coordination of care and seeks to enable the individual to make sense of their experience of illness and disease within the setting of their particular life history.[8] By all these means general practice endeavours to resist the medicalisation of illness in a way which should parallel the way in which primary care resists the medicalisation of health. General practice, with its focus on the needs of the sick individual, and the World Health Organisation's vision of primary care, focused on the health needs of the community, are essentially complementary.

If general practice and primary care are treated as synonymous, both are weakened. An emphasis on general practice medicalises and enfeebles primary care, underestimating and undermining the capacity of individuals and communities to improve their own health. General practitioners and primary health care teams are made to feel responsible for the health of communities when in reality the most powerful determinants of that health lie well beyond their influence. Equally, an emphasis on the primary care of populations marginalises and undervalues the entirely appropriate focus of general practice expertise on the care of individual patients who feel ill.

The strengths of general practice

The root of the well recognised cost effectiveness of the UK system of general practice lies not only in the role of gatekeeper to specialist care, but, more powerfully, in the work which goes on at the interface between illness and disease. By working with the individual patient to distinguish illness caused by unhappiness from that caused by disease, patients can be enabled to benefit from medical science without being needlessly exposed to its considerable dangers[9] It is this aspect of the work of general practice which allows practitioners their most privileged access to their patients and to as much of their experience of life, suffering, endurance and survival as the patient wishes to share.

This brings the powerful internal rewards (see Chapter 1) which, if more widely recognised and valued, have the potential to reverse the sapping of morale which has followed the previous relentless emphasis on the external rewards brought by financial incentives (see Chapter 4). It is perhaps significant that the theoretical underpinning of the core tasks of general practice was articulated during the two decades which followed the 1965 Charter for General Practice at a time when general practice was relatively sheltered from the attention of policymakers and politicians.

The accelerating pace of change over the last decade, apparently unmodified by the recent change of government, has seemed to threaten many of the core tasks of general practice,[10] and damage the morale of general practitioners.[11] Current talk of charges for general practitioner services promises to further erode the equity of access to which the NHS has always been committed.

Experience in other European countries shows that patient charges also profoundly effect the dynamics of the consultation and undermine the ability of the practitioner to use time as a tool.[12] This demonstrates how easily the effectiveness of general practice could be impaired by policy changes which seek to modify the workings of general practice without the prerequisite understanding.

Another danger is the pressure on general practitioners to assume a public health role (through commissioning and purchasing) and a population perspective, which undervalues both the primacy of the general practice focus on illness, and the substantial contribution to the greater public health which is made by general practitioners and other members of primary health care teams in a series of encounters with sick individuals.

The primary health care team as a bridge

In contrast, and contrary to much contemporary rhetoric, the central tasks of general practice are in no way undermined by the

63

developing role of the other primary health care disciplines. Over recent years we have been constantly exhorted to provide a seamless service to patients which has seemed to imply that there should be no overlap between the roles of the different disciplines. We might do well to remember that seams are designed to hold things together and we should not worry that the roles of practice nurse and general practitioner, or health visitor and district nurse, seem to overlap.

It is inevitable that different disciplines will share experience and expertise, and such sharing holds the work of teams together. It is for this reason that it is more helpful to think in terms of interdisciplinary rather than multidisciplinary working and education. An interdisciplinary approach implies the recognition of both common and distinct areas of expertise and makes devising and defining ways of working effectively together an explicit part of the learning and practice agenda.[13] The enormous scope for interdisciplinary education within practice teams who already share learning situations grounded in real practice is currently impeded by the processes by which each profession accredits its own members' education separately. There is an urgent need to develop a system for the joint or independent accreditation of team learning.

Teams have the potential to forge links between general practice and the broader concept of primary care, and between health services and their users and communities. Health visitors, most recently the most unjustly maligned and undervalued members of the primary care team, probably have the most to offer. Trained as public health nurses, they bring a population based public health perspective to their work with practice teams but, too often, unrealistic caseloads and health visitors' statutory responsibilities for children under five mean that they are prevented from using and developing their skills. Primary care teams are slowly being offered more opportunities to work closely with social workers seconded from local authority departments and this extends the possibilities of building bridges with local communities.

The voluntary sector offers similar scope but much depends on whether both the primary care team and the voluntary sector organisation can muster sufficient resources, of both time and personnel, to build effective networks. As ever, the inverse care law[14] applies, and the greater a practice population's need for social support, the less is its community able to offer, and the more overstretched are all the local agencies, impairing effective liaison and joint working. The legacy of the previous administration is a learned helplessness in the face of the socioeconomic determinants of health and a distorted concept of health promotion. Both must be overcome.

The focus on the development of general practice has distracted attention from what could be achieved by pursuing the World Health Organisation's model of primary care and community development. The limited amount of work which has been undertaken in the UK shows that local communities are fully aware of the wider determinants of their health, and prioritise improvements to housing, transport and employment, and the provision of safe play areas for children.[15]

General practitioners and other primary health care workers place high value on resources provided by local communities offering social support and leisure and educational opportunities.[16] The recent proposal that the lottery should be used to fund a network of Healthy Living Centres[17] could provide the basis for building a World Health Organisation model of primary care in the UK,[18] although it is hard to see how these initiatives will be sustained in deprived areas if only start up funding is to be provided.

The health service is part of the good society and both promote health

The renewed emphasis on the rights and responsibilities of citizens offers the possibility of moving on from the reductionist view of the patient as a consumer. Seeing beyond the individual patient to the fellow citizen supports the model of doctor and patient working together as coproducers of health, each bringing different types of knowledge and expertise to the consultation.[19] These consultations involve dialogue and storytelling which have both a clinical and a social dimension,[20] and so reflect the wider relationship between health and society.

Successive consultations with individual patients are the building blocks by which general practitioners forge powerful links with their local communities. Joint working with other professional colleagues in primary health care teams vastly extends the range of expertise and interventions which can be offered to patients.[21] If such teams can be sited within, form part of, and contribute towards vibrant, stable, and cohesive communities then we will begin to see general practice operating as an essential component of a much broader programme of primary health care[22] and we will begin to create a wholly healthier nation.

1. Galbraith JK. *The Good Society. The Humane Agenda.* London: Sinclair-Stevenson, 1996.
2. NHS Executive. *Priorities and planning guidance: 1996/7.* Wetherby: Department of Health, 1995.
3. Gunnell DJ, Peters TJ, Kammerling RM, Brooks J. Relation between parasuicide, suicide, psychiatric admissions, and socioeconomic deprivation. *Br Med J* 1995; **311**: 226-30.
4. Bunker JP, Stansfield S, Potter J. Freedom, responsibility, and health. *Br Med J* 1996; **313**: 1582-5.
5. Rudebeck CE. General practice and the dialogue of clinical practice. *Scand J Prim Health Care* 1991, Supplement 1.
6. WHO. *Primary Health Care: Report of the International Conference on Primary Health Care, Alma Ata, USSR (Health for All Series, No. 1).* Geneva: World Health Organisation, 1978.
7. Heath I. *The mystery of general practice.* London: The Nuffield Provincial Hospitals Trust, 1995.
8. Toon P. *What is good general practice?* Occasional paper 65. Exeter: RCGP, 1994.
9. Barsky AJ, Borus JF. Somatization and medicalization in the era of managed care. *JAMA* 1995; **274**: 1931-34.
10. Stott NCH. When something is good, more of the same is not always better. *Br J Gen Pract* 1993; **43**: 254-258.
11. Sutherland UJ, Cooper CJ. Job stress, satisfaction and mental health among general practitioners before and after the introduction of a new contract. *Br Med J* 1992; **304**: 1545-1548.
12. Fry J, Horder J. *Primary health care in an international context.* London: The Nuffield Provincial Hospitals Trust, 1994.
13. CAIPE. *Principles of interprofessional education.* London: UK centre for the Advancement of Interprofessional Education, 1996.
14. Hart JT. The inverse care law. *Lancet* 1971; **i** 405-412.
15. Murray SA, Tapson J, Turnbull L, McCallum J, Little A. Listening to local voices: adapting rapid appraisal to assess health and social needs in general practice. *Br Med J* 1994; **308**: 698-700
16. Lorentzon M, Jarman B, Bajekal M. *Report of the inner City Task Force of the Royal College of General Practitioners* (Occasional Paper 66). Exeter: Royal College of General Practitioners, 1994.
17. Secretary of State for Culture, Media and Sport. *The people's lottery* (Cm 3709). London, 1997
18. Green J, Prince D. *"It's called a health project... but they do a bit of all sorts there". An evaluation of the Riverside Community Health Project.* Newcastle: Social welfare Research Unit, University of Northumbria, 1996.
19. Hart JT. *Feasible socialism: the National Health Service, past, present and future.* London: Socialist Health Association, 1994.
20. Kleinman A. *The illness narratives: suffering, healing and the human condition.* New York: Basic Books, 1988.
21. Kendrick T, Hilton S. Broader teamwork in primary care. *Br Med J* 1997; **36**: 672-5.
22. Vuori H. Health for all, primary health care and general practitioners. *J Roy Coll Gen Pract* 1986; **36**: 398-402.

INDEX